BARBITURATES

Drug Abuse And Alcoholism Series

BARBITURATES: THEIR USE, MISUSE, AND ABUSE

By
Donald R. Wesson, M.D., and
David E. Smith, M.D.

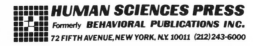

HUMAN SCIENCES PRESS
Formerly *BEHAVIORAL PUBLICATIONS INC.*
72 FIFTH AVENUE, NEW YORK, N.Y. 10011 (212) 243-6000

Library of Congress Catalog Number 76-41079

ISBN: 0-87705-249-2

Copyright © 1977 by Human Sciences Press
72 Fifth Avenue, New York, New York 10011

Printed in the United States of America
6789   987654321
Library of Congress Cataloging in Publication Data

Wesson, Donald R
    Barbiturates, their use, misuse, and abuse.

    Bibliography: p.
    Includes index.
    1. Barbiturates. 2. Drug abuse. I. Smith, David
Elvin, 1939-   joint author. II. Title. [DNLM:
1. Barbiturates—Therapeutic use. 2. Barbiturates—
Poisoning. 3. Drug abuse. 4. Drug dependence. QV88
W515b]
RC568.B3W47   615'.782   76-41079
ISBN 0-87705-249-2

CONTENTS

PREFACE

Our interest in barbiturates was stimulated in 1968 when we became involved with treating increasing numbers of individuals who were either physically dependent on barbiturates or experiencing medical complications following barbiturate abuse. Following the "Summer of Love" in 1967, amphetamines and barbiturates began to replace psychedelics as the dominant drugs used in the Haight-Ashbury district of San Francisco, and increasing numbers of individuals were treated at the Haight-Ashbury Free Medical Clinic for complications following barbiturate use. Some individuals took primarily barbiturates—either orally or intravenously—others used barbiturates to terminate a "run" with illicitly manufactured intravenous methamphetamine called "crystal."

Later, barbiturates were replaced largely by heroin, although many heroin users turned to barbiturates when their supply of heroin was low or exhausted. Other individuals whose life-styles were dedicated to drug use but who were unable to compete successfully in the highly competitive heroin marketplace, primarily used barbiturates and only rarely heroin.

Because of our growing reputation for treating barbiturate abusers, other physicians and treatment agencies consulted us or referred barbiturate abusers to us. We also became aware of another population of users who were not associated with the drug scene among youth in the Haight-Ashbury. These individuals obtained their drugs from physicians and came to our attention because of chronic intoxication or after an overdose.

In 1973 individuals within the Special Action Office for Drug Abuse Prevention became interested in the abuse of drugs other than heroin. This interest was manifested in the development of a series of Polydrug Demonstration and Research Projects. The first project was established in San Francisco. Our involvement in these projects allowed us to extend our research into barbiturate abuse and to compare observations and treatment experiences with other individuals throughout the country.

We soon became convinced of the need for a pragmatically oriented, clinical book focusing on the barbiturates— their current medical uses as well as misuse and abuse. As we compiled the literature, we began to appreciate the complexity and enormity of our task.

Important contributions to the literature on barbiturates are scattered throughout the journals of anesthesia, psychiatry, drug abuse, pharmacology, and general medicine. Although the literature is now too voluminous to be listed or even comprehensively reviewed in one book, we have attempted to bring together the information and references of greatest importance to health professionals. Whenever possible, we reviewed original sources to reduce to a minimum the errors that inevitably occur when secondary sources are used. Except for the early literature, which was written almost exclusively in German, we reviewed only the English language literature. We critiqued case reports in terms of the rationality of their conclusions and have included in the bibliography and references citations of original case reports and reviews which are readily accessible or especially useful. Many of the case reports we studied were discarded because their findings were based on tenuous cause-and-effect relationships. For example, clinical studies reporting morphological changes in brain tissue secondary to chronic ingestion of barbiturates failed to take into account the degree to which these changes were the result of hypoxia or other illnesses. Experimental studies were evaluated in terms of methodology, statistical analysis, and conclusions. In some cases, we recomputed the statistics contained in these studies to satisfy ourselves that the authors' conclusions were valid.

We included classical studies, reports of new developments, and articles that provided useful overviews of selected topics. Of special note are the following: Lundy's and Osterberg's review (1929) of the literature on the chemistry, pharmacology, and clinical use of the derivatives of barbituric acid, and Tatum's discussion (1939) about the barbiturate problem that existed in the late 1930s. Wulff's monograph (1959) is an outstanding review of the medical aspects of barbiturate withdrawal.

The results of much of the early analytical work are of questionable accuracy when compared with findings that were obtained after technology had advanced to the point where it was possible to make practical more specific identification of compounds. Although analytical methodology is of great importance, the clinician is interested primarily in results. Therefore, we have omitted discussion of procedural methodology. Similarly, we did not thoroughly review the use of barbiturates as anesthetic agents or as adjuncts to anesthesia—a topic that has been reviewed extensively in *Intravenous Anaesthesia* by J. W. Dundee and G. M. Wyant (1974).

Because our primary focus in this book is the clinical application of barbiturates and drug abuse, we included reviews of animal studies only when the data's clinical usefulness was apparent. In attempting to synthesize our material into one volume, we hope we have achieved more than a modicum of success in providing health professionals and other interested individuals with a balanced and rational perspective on the use, misuse, and abuse of barbiturates.

We gratefully acknowledge the efforts of those who assisted us during the writing and editing of this book. Laurie Linda provided research and editorial assistance during the early stages of the book's development. Debbie Slutsky typed numerous drafts and provided many helpful stylistic suggestions, Leslie Simon provided editorial coordination of the final stages, and Grace Dammann provided valuable library research assistance. Elizabeth Bowman edited the book and greatly improved its readability and organization.

While writing this book, we were involved with the National Polydrug Projects funded by the Division of Resource Development of the National Institute on Drug Abuse. Barbiturates, alone or in combination, were found to be the most commonly abused prescription drug nationally in all the projects—a fact that provided additional impetus and resources for us to complete this volume.

Chapter 1

INTRODUCTION

When barbiturates were introduced into the field of medicine in 1903, they were a technological improvement over the bromides, which at the time were the most commonly prescribed sedatives. Like most technological achievements, this discovery had both malevolent and benevolent consequences. The availability of barbiturates for treatment of anxiety and insomnia has improved the quality of life for hundreds of thousands of individuals throughout the world. In addition, barbiturates are important adjuncts to surgical anesthesia, and phenobarbital is still the drug of first choice in the treatment of many patients with major motor seizures.

These benefits notwithstanding, barbiturates—especially secobarbital and pentobarbital—have become the most common drugs of abuse after alcohol and tobacco, involving more individuals than the widely publicized heroin epidemic. And, as described later, barbiturates are capable of producing physical dependence that is of greater medical consequence than opiate dependency.

Although the bulk of this book is devoted to the physiological and medical aspects of barbiturate use and abuse, we have also attempted to develop a broad overview of the social, political, and economic aspects of the topic. As a result, much of the information will be of value not only to medical students, physicians, and other health professionals but to social workers, psychologists, attorneys, and legislators who are interested in the field of drug abuse.

Physicians and medical students who are concerned about appropriate prescription of barbiturates and other sedative-hypnotics should find the basic pharmacological information reviewed in Chapter 2 especially helpful. All readers, however, should find the majority of the chapter useful because it describes the symptoms and effects of both acute toxicity and chronic usage.

An understanding of the medical uses for barbiturates is important for health professionals who provide direct services. This information is contained in Chapter 3. Social workers and psychologists often consult us because they are concerned about a patient's barbiturate "abuse." On examination, however, we are obliged to point out to them that these patients are using the drugs under medical supervision in reasonable dosages for appropriate clinical indications. All professionals who are interested in the problem of drug abuse should find Chapter 4 of interest because it defines misuse and abuse and describes the various patterns of barbiturate abuse.

Chapters 5 and 6 offer specific recommendations for medical treatment of the complications of barbiturate abuse—e.g., chronic and episodic intoxication, overdose, withdrawal symptoms, and physical dependency—as well as a general understanding of a variety of treatment techniques ranging from management of overdose to appropriate detoxification procedures and aftercare treatment modalities.

Chapter 7 covers several nonmedical aspects of barbiturate abuse, such as the availability and sources of drugs of abuse and the social and economic factors involved in drug abuse. The following brief history summarizes the early development of barbiturates.

Barbiturates comprise a class of chemical compounds that are derivatives of barbituric acid, which was first synthesized by Nobel Prize-winning German chemist Adolph Baeyer in 1863. Accounts vary with regard to how barbituric acid (Barbitursäure) acquired its name. According to *The Origin of Medical Terms* (Skinner, 1970), the compound was named after a Munich waitress named Barbara who contributed urine samples for analysis at the Baeyer chemical factory in Leverkusen, Germany. Wain (1958) suggests, however, that the compound was called barbituric acid because it was synthesized on St. Barbara's Day.

In 1882 Conrad and Guthzeit synthesized 5,5-diethylbarbituric acid (barbital), the first barbiturate used for medical purposes. Twenty-one years later, Emile Fischer, a student of Baeyer's who also received a Nobel Prize in chemistry, and Baron Joseph von Mering (1903) introduced barbital into clinical medicine under the trade name of Veronal—a name derived from the Italian city of Verona. (The generic product is called barbital in the United States, barbitone in England, and barbituric acid in Germany). A year later, Fischer and Dilthey (1904) prepared a series of barbiturates and thiobarbiturate analogs. Fischer synthesized phenylethylbarbituric acid, known by the trade name of Luminal or the generic name of phenobarbital. Its use was described by Loewe (1912), Juliusburger (1912), Impens (1912), and Geissler (1912). That same year, Hauptmann (1912) reported the anticonvulsant properties of phenobarbital, and a patent was issued for commercial synthesis of phenobarbital. Juliusburger (1914) described the use of diallylbarbituric acid (Dial®) as a sedative and hypnotic in psychosis as well as for morphine and alcohol withdrawal.

World War I stimulated American interest in the manufacture of phenobarbital. Rising and Stieglitz (1918) described an alternative synthesis to the patented process for phenobarbital in the *Journal of the American Chemical Society,* and by 1920 barbiturates were widely used. In 1922 Klaesi, a Swiss psychiatrist, introduced "continuous sleep therapy" using Somnifen, a mixture of diethylbarbituric acid and diallylbarbituric acid. Dox and Yoder (1922) of Parke, Davis and Company reported on the synthesis and hypnotic properties of 5-n-butyl-5-ethylbarbituric acid. A year later, Shonle and Moment (1923) of Eli Lilly and Company synthesized and defined the biological activity of a series of additional barbiturates, including isoamylethylbarbituric acid (amobarbital) and *sec*-butylethylbarbituric acid (butabarbital). By 1929 amobarbital was used clinically as a hypnotic, and Bleckwenn (1930) advocated using intravenous injections of sodium amobarbital to induce sleep in patients suffering acute mania, catatonic schizophrenia, and acute delirium; he also reported that status epilepticus could be controlled with amobarbital. Secobarbital was synthesized in 1930 by Shonle, Keltch, and Swanson. In 1935 Tabern and Volwiler synthesized Pentothal® (thiopental) and Lundy (1935) introduced it as an intravenous anesthetic the same year. Fentothal® was marketed as an intravenous anesthetic in the United States by 1936.

Most barbiturates commonly used today have been in clinical use for more than 50 years. So far, the benzodiazepines (Valium®, librium®, Tranxene®, Serax®, Clonopin®, and Dalmane®) represent the only effective challenge to the barbiturates.

Many details of the barbiturates' mechanism of action and metabolism are still unknown, despite wide clinical usage. In the early 1970s, studies in sleep laboratories began to challenge the efficacy of barbiturates for inducing sleep for more than a few nights and also provided a physiological basis for determining why many individuals became dependent on barbiturates (e.g., Evans et al., 1968; Kales et al., 1974).

Chapter 2

PHARMACOLOGICAL CHARACTERISTICS OF THE BARBITURATES

Barbituric acid, the compound from which the barbiturates are derived, is a fusion of urea and malonic acid (Baeyer, 1863). The net result of the reactions, which actually involve intermediate products, is shown in Figure 2.1.

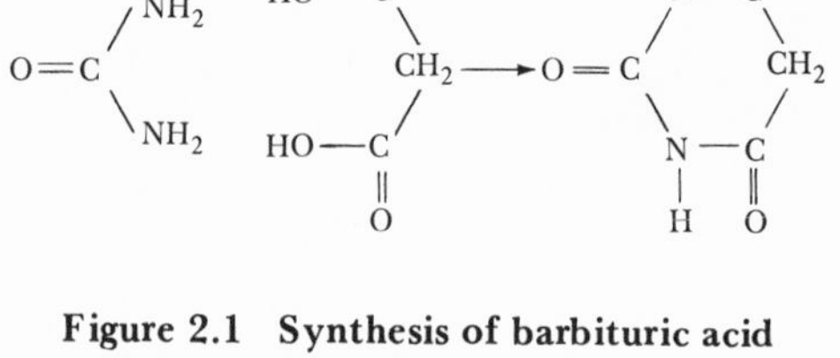

Figure 2.1   Synthesis of barbituric acid

Barbituric acid (Figure 2.2) has no effect on the central nervous system (CNS). Barbiturates are pyrimidine ring derivatives. The pyrimidine ring occurs in many other biologically important compounds, such as Vitamin B_1 (thiamine) and the nucleic acids cytosine, uracil, and thymine (see Figure 2.2B). CNS-active barbiturates have various carbon chains at positions three and five. Enclosing a ring at positions C4 and C5 with radicals containing nitrogen creates the purine structure, which also occurs in nucleic acids, vitamins, and CNS-active drugs such as caffeine (see Figure 2.2C). The thiobarbiturates thiopental (Pentothal®) and thiamylal (Surital®) have a sulfa radical attached to C2 in place of oxygen.

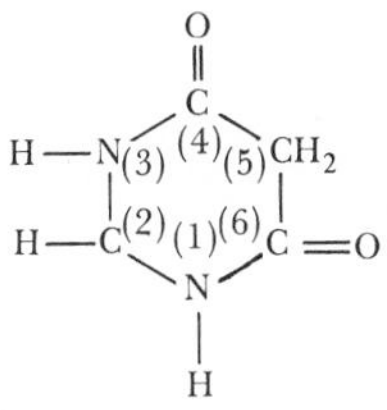

A. Barbituric acid

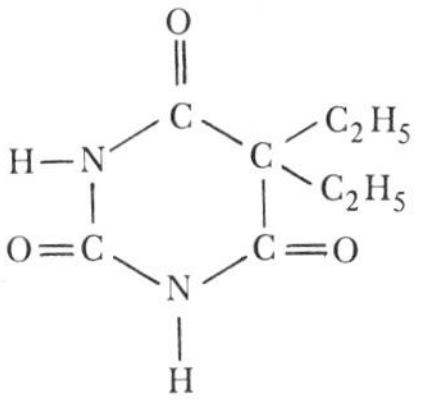

Barbital

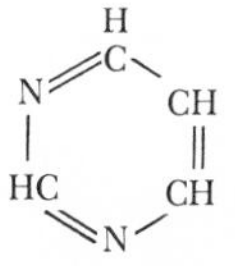

B. Pyrimidine nucleus

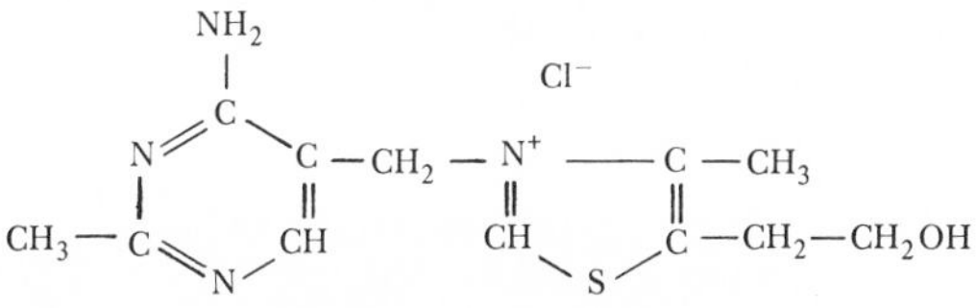

Thiamine hydrochloride

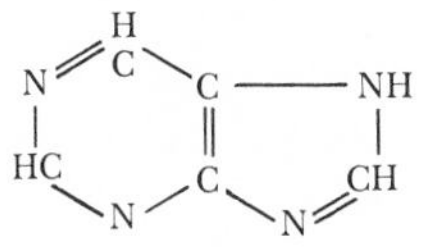

C. Purine nucleus

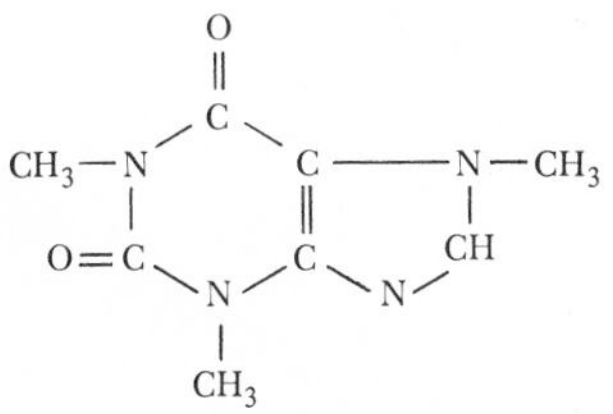

Caffeine

Figure 2.2 Comparison of chemical structures.
A. Barbituric acid and one of its derivatives, barbital.
B. Pyrimidine nucleus and thiamine hydrochloride.
C. Purine nucleus and caffeine.

As the number of carbon atoms attached to C5 increases, sedative properties increase until seven carbon atoms are reached. Additional carbon atoms reduce the sedative properties. Branched aliphatic groups attached to C5 are more active and less toxic than the straight chains, and barbiturates with dissimilar alkyl radicals are more active than symmetrically substituted ones. Although the addition of unsaturated radicals increases the sedative properties of the barbiturates, convulsive properties also appear (Meyer & Rollet, 1964). The propensity of some barbiturates to induce convulsions is greatly increased by the addition of allyl groups at the 1-nitrogen position. The convulsive barbiturates are not used clinically.

Although more than 2,000 barbiturates have been synthesized, only about a dozen are commonly used clinically. Table 2.1 lists the generic name, trade name, and chemical structure of commonly prescribed barbiturates, which are subdivided according to the pharmacological duration of action of a single dose.

This classical arrangement of the barbiturates was developed by Fitch (1930), who recognized that because of differences in rate of absorption between oral and intravenous administration of the drug, duration of action could be determined most precisely if the drug was administered intravenously. He conceptualized this classification as one that would permit the rational selection of one barbiturate over another for experimental and clinical use. But Fitch's critics point out that he failed to consider variations in duration of action related to dosage. For example, ultra-short-acting anesthetic agents, which Fitch listed as being active for less than three hours, can actually be active for many hours if the dose is large enough. Furthermore, subtle cerebral dysfunction persists far beyond the period of anesthetic action. Following a large overdose of secobarbital or pentobarbital (short-acting barbiturates), an individual may be in coma for several days.

Fitch's classification refers to the duration of action of a single low dose of the drug. The large variation in pharmacological effects in low-dose pharmacokinetics is more closely related to redistribution of the drug within the different body tissues than it is to destruction or excretion. Dundee and Wyant (1974) recommended a classification based on the speed of onset of a drug's action as well as the duration of its effects. For instance, the short-acting barbiturates such as secobarbital, pentobarbital, and amobarbital are used primarily as oral sedatives (but are sometimes administered parenterally) and have a delayed onset of action following intravenous injection. The fast-acting barbiturates, which are used as intravenous anesthetics and have no delay in onset of action, comprise a second group, while the long-acting barbiturates such as phenobarbital form a third.

EFFECTS ON CENTRAL NERVOUS SYSTEM

In clinically useful dosages, the barbiturates' primary site of action is the CNS. These drugs produce depression of the CNS ranging from mild sedation to coma; the degree of depression depends on the type of barbiturate, the amount, the method of administration, and the nervous system's state of excitability.

There is a close correlation between the oil/water partition coefficient and hypnotic potency of the barbiturates. The highly lipid-soluble compounds have the most rapid onset of action—a phenomenon that is probably related to the speed with which they cross the blood-brain barrier (Hansch & Clayton, 1973).

Absorption and Distribution

Barbiturates are distributed by the plasma among the various body organs, muscle, fat, and brain. Organs with a

Table 2.1 Classification of Barbiturates by Duration of Pharmacological Effects of a Single Dose

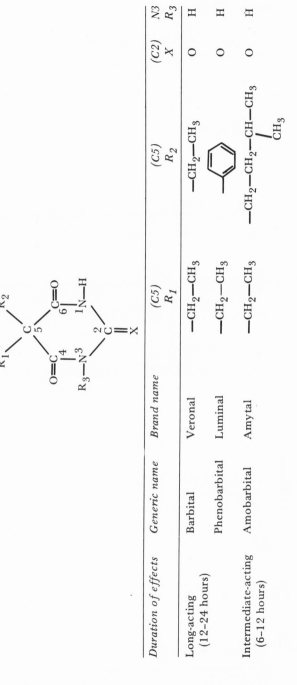

Duration of effects	Generic name	Brand name	(C5) R_1	(C5) R_2	(C2) X	(N3) R_3
Long-acting (12–24 hours)	Barbital	Veronal	—CH$_2$—CH$_3$	—CH$_2$—CH$_3$	O	H
	Phenobarbital	Luminal	—CH$_2$—CH$_3$	⟨benzene ring⟩	O	H
Intermediate-acting (6–12 hours)	Amobarbital	Amytal	—CH$_2$—CH$_3$	—CH$_2$—CH$_2$—CH—CH$_3$ | CH$_3$	O	H

Class	Chemical name	Brand name	R₁	R₂	X	R₃
	Butabarbital	Butisol	$-CH_2-CH_3$	$-CH-CH_2-CH_3$ (CH_3)	O	H
Short-acting (3–6 hours)	Pentobarbital	Nembutal	$-CH_2-CH_3$	$-CH-CH_2-CH_3$ (CH_3)	O	H
	Secobarbital	Seconal	$-CH_2-CH=CH_2$	$-CH-CH_2-CH_3$ (CH_3)	O	H
Ultrashort-acting (15 min.–3 hours)	Thiamylal	Surital (Thioseconal)	$-CH_2-CH=CH_2$	$-CH-CH_2-CH_3$ (CH_3)	S	H
	Thiopental	Pentothal (Intraval)	$-CH_2-CH_3$	$-CH-CH_2-CH_3$ (CH_3)	S	H

higher blood flow take up barbiturates first. After a single intravenous injection of thiopental, for example, the maximum concentrations of the drug in organs and the brain are reached within one minute; uptake in muscle continues for about 15 minutes; and uptake in fat, for 1½ to 2½ hours (Dundee & Wyant, 1974).

Although the barbiturates are well absorbed from the stomach, the short-acting ones absorb more readily than those that are longer acting. Alcohol enhances absorption and produces an additive CNS depression. Solutions containing water-soluble sodium salts of barbiturates can be injected either intramuscularly or intravenously. In solution, these sodium salts—including those prepared by pharmaceutical companies specifically for injection—are highly alkaline. Because barbiturates cross the placental barrier within a few minutes after injection, the concentration in fetal blood quickly approaches that of maternal venous blood.

Barbiturates are bound to varying degrees by serum albumin. The unbound drug in plasma is the physiologically active component. In general, barbiturates with longer side chains at positions 2 and 5 are bound more strongly than are those with short chains. The thiobarbiturates are bound more strongly than the oxybarbiturates. Goldbaum and Smith (1954) studied 17 barbiturates *in vitro* and found that the least amount of binding to serum albumin occurred with barbital (5 per cent) while the greatest amount occurred with thiopental (65 per cent). More recent studies reviewed by Hansch and Clayton (1973) indicate that biological availability is not necessarily a linear function of concentration and is more adequately described by a second order equation.

Metabolism and Excretion

With the exception of barbital and phenobarbital, commonly used barbiturates are transformed in the body into inactive metabolites, primarily by the liver. Three major mechanisms are involved in this degradation process: (1) side-chain oxidation, (2) nitrogen dealkylation, and (3) desulfuration of thiobarbiturates. Some barbiturates utilize more than one of these mechanisms as well as minor metabolic pathways, and side-chain oxidation can occur in several different ways.

Barbiturates that are not metabolized by the liver are excreted unchanged in the urine. Phenobarbital and barbital are dependent mainly on renal excretion: e.g., 65 to 90 per cent of the total amount of phenobarbital ingested appears in the urine unaltered. The other barbiturates appear in the urine in negligible quantities. (See Park, 1971, for a review of biotransformation of barbiturates.)

The duration of the effects of the ultrashort-acting barbiturates listed in Table 2.1 is not related to the drugs' metabolic destruction but to the rate at which they are redistributed throughout the body. For example, approximately 0.3 per cent of a dose of thiopental is excreted unchanged in the urine. Ten to 15 per cent of the dose is metabolized per hour—far too slow a rate to account for the brief action of this compound. How soon a patient will awake after a single anesthetic dose of thiopental depends on how quickly the drug shifts from his brain to other tissues. The rate at which different tissues absorb thiopental is determined by the rate of blood flow. The brain, kidneys, and heart are saturated 30 seconds after intravenous administration, while muscles and skin require 15 to 30 minutes to reach saturation. Therefore, the high concentration absorbed by the brain is then redistributed to muscles, skin, and fat. The resulting drop in the effective concentration in the brain accounts for the extremely short action observed.

Detection in Biological Fluids

Barbiturates can be detected in the urine by thin-layer chromatography, gas chromatography, the free radical-assay technique, or the enzyme-multiplied immunoassay technique. The minimum concentration of barbiturates that can be detected in the urine by these methods ranges from 1 to 3 micrograms per milliliter. Currently, thin-layer chromatography and gas chromatography are the standard methods. When these tests are performed properly, the incidence of false positive results is less than 1 per cent (Catlin, 1973). Barbiturates can be detected in serum extracts by using either gas chromatography or thin-layer chromatography.

Acute Toxicity

IMPAIRED FUNCTIONING.   In a study of acute toxicity using the double-blind technique, Loomis and West (1958) compared the effects of the following drugs on eight adult male subjects who had been trained in simulated driving performance: 100 mg. of secobarbital, 50 mg. of chlorpromazine, 400 mg. of meprobamate, and 300 mg. of phenaglycodol (a placebo was used as a control). The automated driving apparatus measured the parameters of the subjects' reaction time and steering errors. A control test was conducted after the subjects had eaten a light breakfast. The first dose of the drug was then administered orally, and the subjects were tested again after one hour and two hours had elapsed. Two-and-a-half to three hours after the initial medication, they ate a light lunch and received a second oral dose of the drug an hour later. Final driving tests were conducted one hour and two hours after the second dose. Although meprobamate and chlorpromazine impaired the subjects' functioning within the parameters specified for the experiment, secobarbital produced the most significant degree of impairment, which Loomis and West equated with the amount of impairment produced by 150 mg. of alcohol per ml. of blood.

Smith and Beecher (1960) studied 15 male members of college swimming teams who had taken 100 mg. of secobarbital, 14 mg. of amphetamine, or a placebo. Each man swam six times under each of the following conditions: rested-solo, rested-group, fatigued-solo, and fatigued-group. After each trial, each man estimated his performance time and evaluated the quality of his performance in detail. Secobarbital not only impaired the swimmers' performance to a significant degree, it impaired their ability to assess their performance accurately. Under the influence of secobarbital, they believed that they had performed unusually well; in actuality, however, their performance was significantly poorer than usual. Although the investigators found that amphetamines improved the men's performance, the results concerning the drug's effects on their judgment were inconclusive.

The relevance of these studies to patient populations is uncertain. Clinical observation leads us to believe that the motor performance of some extremely anxious patients improves with drug therapy. Also, some of the impairment noted in these single-dose studies would be viewed as transient side effects by clinicians because it tends to disappear after three to seven days of therapy. Whether tranquilizers improve the performance of anxious patients is a question that needs further investigation.

SUBJECTIVE EFFECTS.   Intoxication caused by short-acting barbiturates is qualitatively similar to being drunk on alcohol. Most commonly, individuals self-administer secobarbital or pentobarbital to produce intoxication—an important parameter in the potential for abuse of these drugs. Subjectively, an individual experiences disinhibition as stimulation. When Ideström and Cadenius (1963) gave a group of subjects oral doses of amobarbital and then administered a series of neuropsychiatric tests, they obtained the following results. After doses of 150 mg., the subjects felt more tired and performed less satisfactorily on some neuropsychiatric tests than did subjects who had taken 300 mg.

However, the performance of subjects who ingested 450 mg. was more severely impaired than the performance of subjects who had taken 150 or 300 mg. or a placebo.

The effects of barbiturate intoxication may vary, even in the same individual. The user's *expectations* have a marked influence on the drug's effect. For instance, the person who takes 200 mg. of secobarbital and expects to fall asleep will usually sleep, if provided with a suitable environment. Another individual, who takes the same amount of secobarbital and expects to have a good time in a stimulating environment, may experience a state of para-doxical stimulation or disinhibition euphoria. For example it is not uncommon for individuals to ingest two capsules (200 mg.) of secobarbital at a rock concert and achieve a state of intoxication that is similar to that produced by ingesting 60 to 120 ml. of alcohol.

Disinhibition euphoria is not necessarily synonymous with intoxication; the affective mood associated with in-toxication may vary widely, depending on the individual, the drug, the dosage, the surroundings, and expectations. Individuals intoxicated with phenobarbital commonly ex-hibit an unsteady gait, slurred speech, sustained vertical and horizontal nystagmus, and poor judgment, but they often describe their subjective state as unpleasant or dys-phoric. Furthermore, a person's perception of intoxication caused by any drug as pleasant is in part a learned response and is influenced to a large extent by his expectations and the environment in which he happens to be at the time.

The disinhibition euphoria produced by the barbitu-rates and certain other sedative-hypnotics makes them ap-pealing as intoxicants. In general, disinhibition is directly related to hypnotic potency. The concentrations of barbitu-rates that correlate with different behavioral changes are shown in Table 2.2. Note that there is appreciable variation among the different barbiturates in terms of the blood con-

Table 2.2   Expected Behavioral Changes in Nontolerant Individuals, Related to Concentration of Barbiturates in the Blood

Type of barbiturate	*Concentration (mg./ml.)*	*Expected changes in behavior*
Pentobarbital	0.5 to 3.0	Therapeutic range: sedated, calm, relaxed and easily aroused.
	10 to 15	Comatose.
	15 to 40	Usual lethal levels.
Secobarbital	0.5 to 5.0	Therapeutic range: sedated, calm, relaxed and easily aroused.
	10 to 15	Comatose.
	15 to 40	Usual lethal levels.
Amobarbital	2 to 10	Therapeutic range: sedated, calm, relaxed and easily aroused.
	30 to 40	Comatose.
	40 to 80	Usual lethal levels.
Butabarbital	3 to 25	Therapeutic range: sedated, calm, relaxed and easily aroused.
	40 to 60	Comatose.
	60 to 100	Usual lethal levels.
Phenobarbital	5 to 40	Therapeutic range: sedated, calm, relaxed and easily aroused.
	50 to 80	Comatose.
	100 to 200	Usual lethal levels.

Source: Adapted from Parker et al., 1970, p. 143.

centrations required for therapeutic purposes and to produce intoxication. There are also considerable variations between individuals in response to a particular blood level.

Intoxication reduces an individual's ability to make accurate judgments and may markedly impair motor coordination. The relative ability of barbiturates and other sedative-hypnotics to produce disinhibition euphoria is compared in Table 2.3.

Table 2.3   Estimated Ability of Common Sedative-Hypnotics to Produce Disinhibition Euphoria

Common generic name	Common trade names	Estimated ability to produce disinhibition euphoria[a]
Alcohol	Many brand names	++++
Amobarbital	Amytal	+++
Butabarbital	Butisol	++
Chloral Hydrate	Aquachloral Supprettes, Felsules, Kessodrate, Noctec, Rectules, Somnos	++
Chlordiazepoxide HCl	Libritabs, Librium	++
Diazepam	Valium	+++
Flurazepam HCl	Dalmane	+
Glutethimide	Doriden	+++
Meprobamate	Equanil, Kesso-Bamate, Meprospan, Meprotabs, Miltown, SK-Bamate	+++
Methaqualone	Optimil, Parest, Quaalude, Somnafac, Sopor	++++
Methyprylen	Noludar	+++
Pentobarbital	Nembutal	++++
Phenobarbital	Eskabarb, Luminal, Solfoton, Stental	+
Secobarbital	Seco-8, Seconal	++++
Secobarbital and Amobarbital	Tuinal	++++

[a]+ = slight tendency to produce disinhibition euphoria; ++++ = strong tendency to produce disinhibition euphoria.
Source: Adapted from Wesson and Smith, 1973, p. 88.

EFFECT ON THE EEG.   In the conscious individual, barbiturates produce an increase in amplitude and frequency of the EEG. This can be observed in Figure 2.3. The dominant frequency is typically 15 to 30 Hertz (Hz). This activation appears first in the frontal leads and spreads to the occipital and parietal cortex as the dosage is increased. At dosages that produce unconsciousness, the EEG shows large-amplitude slow waves of two to eight Hz. As the dosage is increased even further, brief periods of electrical silence appear. In extreme overdose, all electrical activity ceases. This is one case in which a "flat" EEG cannot be equated with clinical death, and the effects are fully reversible unless hypoxic damage occurs. Thus the physician should consider the possibility of barbiturate intoxication, even in cases that appear to involve trauma. In a patient whose head had been injured in an automobile accident, we

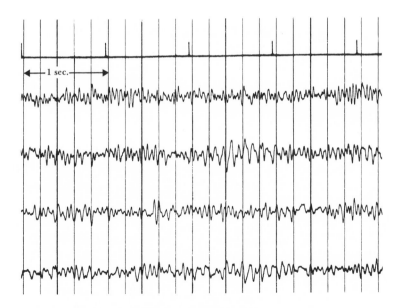

Figure 2.3   EEG showing fast-wave activity produced by barbiturate intoxication.

observed a flat EEG and found an extremely high concentration of barbiturates in his blood. He was maintained on a life-support system in an intensive care unit and recovered.

Side Effects of Oral Doses

When used orally in recommended doses, the barbiturates are generally nontoxic. Idiosyncratic responses include a variety of allergic reactions. Rashes are not characteristic; they may be urticarial, purpuric, morbilliform, or exfoliative and can involve any part of the body, including mucosal surfaces. The literature contains numerous reports of barbital dermatitis. As early as 1903, Lilienfeld noted that barbital could cause erythema. In 1908 Ormsby described a patient who developed dermatitis and severe systemic reaction five days after taking 0.6 gm. of barbital per day. She developed a fever of 104° to 106° F, delirium, and dermatitis over her entire body. Desquamation took place and her nails turned black and became brittle. She eventually recovered.

In 1918, Luce and Feigl described a case of exanthemas caused by phenobarbital. By 1925 it was recognized that individuals who had sensitivity reactions to one barbiturate were likely to be sensitive to all barbiturates (Vallery-Radot & Blamoutier, 1925). Menninger (1928) estimated that sensitivity reactions occurred in 1 to 3 per cent of patients receiving barbital and phenobarbital. In 1929 Poole studied 11 additional cases and found that four involved cutaneous reactions alone while seven involved both cutaneous and systemic reactions. One fatal case showed bronchial mucosa necrosis, sloughing, and nephritis in addition to cutaneous desquamation. In 1936 Birch reported a case of jaundice related to phenobarbital, and subsequently, a number of fatalities related to phenobarbital sensitivity were described by Sexton, Pike, and Nielson (1941); Welton (1950); and others.

CHRONIC USAGE

Because of tissue accumulation, the pharmacodynamics of chronic doses of barbiturates differ from those that characterize the single dose. The effects of chronic usage have not been studied as thoroughly as have the effects of short-term use. Mental signs of chronic intoxication include confusion, poor judgment, irritability, insomnia, and somatic complaints. Some individuals become emotionally labile. Because chronic barbiturate users generally fail to recognize the relationship between the symptoms of intoxication and their use of barbiturates, if given a choice they will usually opt for more barbiturates.

When Wikler et al. (1955) studied the EEGs of 14 severely intoxicated patients for several weeks, they found that the majority of recordings indicated mixed fast (18 to 25 Hz) and slow (4 to 7 Hz) activity. Some of these patients, however, had normal EEGs despite the fact that in clinical terms they were intoxicated.

Dependency and Tolerance

Barbiturates are capable of producing both physical and psychological dependence and tolerance. Physical dependence refers to the development of objective signs of withdrawal when a patient is deprived of the drug abruptly. The term psychological dependence refers to a strong desire to experience the effects of the drug repeatedly, even in the absence of physical dependence. Tolerance means that the body adapts to the drug and thus larger doses are required to produce the original effects. Table 2.4 compares our estimates concerning the parameters of physical dependence and tolerance of several intoxicants.

Tolerance to barbiturates is of two types: *drug disposition tolerance,* which develops when drug-metabolizing enzyme systems in the liver are activated to destroy

Table 2.4 Parameters of Dependence and Tolerance of
Selected Intoxicants[a]

Drug	Tolerance	Psychological dependence[b]	Physical dependence[b]
Alcohol	+	+++	+++
Pentobarbital	++	+++	+++
Secobarbital	++	+++	+++
Heroin	+++	++++	++++
Marijuana	0	++	0[c]

[a] + = slight degree, ++++ = marked degree.
[b] Refers to how quickly dependence develops rather than to its severity.
[c] Some investigators believe that tetrahydrocannabinol (THC) in dosages greater than 200 mg. per day may produce physical dependence.

barbiturates, and *pharmacodynamic tolerance,* which means that the CNS adapts to the drug's presence. As tolerance to barbiturates develops, the amount needed to maintain the same level of intoxication increases; tolerance to a fatal dosage, however, does not increase more than two-fold. As this occurs, the margin between an intoxicating dosage and a fatal dosage becomes smaller. This phenomenon is illustrated in Figure 2.4.

Cross tolerance refers to the ability of one drug to produce tolerance to another. Barbiturates, alcohol, and other sedative-hypnotics are all cross tolerant. For example, tolerance to alcohol will also produce a tolerance to barbiturates, but the barbiturates are not cross tolerant with opiates and marijuana.

Because of their additive effects, a combination of barbiturates and alcohol may seriously impair one's driving performance, even when the concentration of alcohol in the blood is lower than the amount legally defined as producing intoxication. Therefore, when an individual is intoxicated to a degree that is radically disproportionate to the amount of alcohol in his blood, the concurrent use of barbiturates should be suspected. Because the lethal dose of a barbiturate is far less if alcohol is also ingested, the total amount of depressant present must be considered when evaluating a patient who has attempted suicide.

When under the influence of small doses of barbiturates or a combination of alcohol and barbiturates, a person may "forget" he has already taken barbiturates and continue to ingest them until he reaches a lethal dose. These individuals are described as lacking suicidal intent. This behavior, first mentioned by Richards (1934), has been called drug automatism. Although there have been many references to automatism in the literature (e.g., Locket & Angus, 1952; Long, 1960; Tatum, 1939), the concept is not universally accepted. Dorpat (1974), for ex-

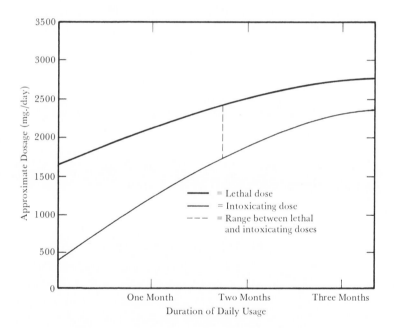

Figure 2.4   Relative relationships between lethal and intoxicating doses of short-acting barbiturates in the blood as tolerance develops. (Dosages are only approximate because of individual differences in tolerance to the drug and patterns of use.)

ample, attributed the amnesia and denial of suicidal intent to the patients' need to deny their self-destructiveness. (See also Jansson, 1961).

Birth Defects

According to the Food and Drug Administration (1974), the use of diphenylhydantoin (Dilantin®) or phenobarbital to control epilepsy is associated with a roughly twofold increase in the incidence of birth defects. The causality of phenobarbital has not been demonstrated unequivocally, however. Other factors, such as the seizure disorder itself, may play a role in fetal abnormalities. The FDA report concluded that "anticonvulsant medication should not be discontinued in pregnant epileptic women in whom the medication is necessary for the prevention of major seizures." Because discontinuing or decreasing the amount of anticonvulsant needed to control seizures increases the risk of status epilepticus in the mother as well as hypoxia in both the mother and fetus and because the majority of epileptic mothers who are treated with anticonvulsant drugs bear normal children, the continuation of drug therapy during pregnancy is considered to involve less risk.

INTERACTION WITH OTHER DRUGS

Barbiturates have the capacity to alter the effects of other drugs by interfering with their absorption or increasing their rate of metabolism or by additive or synergistic effects with the second drug. For example, when barbiturates are taken with opiates, alcohol, or other CNS depressants, the additive respiratory depression can be lethal. Overdoses of multiple drugs are commonly observed in emergency rooms, and in many cases, knowledge of the combined effects of the drugs is important for adequate case management.

Oral Anticoagulants. Phenobarbital, butabarbital, secobarbital, and amobarbital cause a significant decrease in the response to coumarin anticoagulants. This interaction is well documented and is of sufficient magnitude to be of clinical concern. A patient who takes a barbiturate and a coumarin anticoagulant runs the risk of hemorrhage if the dosage of anticoagulant is not decreased when he stops taking the barbiturate. The mechanism of this action is believed to involve the ability of barbiturates to interfere with gastrointestinal absorption of anticoagulants and to induce the production of hepatic microsomal enzymes, which results in increased metabolism of the coumarin anticoagulants (Hansten, 1972). This effect has not been observed with the benzodiazepines (Breckenridge & Orme, 1973).

Diphenylhydantoin (Dilantin®). Because it induces production of hepatic microsomal enzymes, phenobarbital can increase the destruction of diphenylhydantoin. In high dosages, phenobarbital may inhibit the metabolism of diphenylhydantoin. The usual observed effect is an increase in the destruction of diphenylhydantoin, particularly if phenobarbital is added afterward. The effect depends on the patient's previous exposure to enzyme inducers. For optimal management of seizures, the clinician may need to determine the levels of both phenobarbital and diphenylhydantoin in the patient's blood.

Antibiotics. Phenobarbital, when given concomitantly with doxycycline therapy, shortens the half-life of the antibiotic (Neuvonen & Penttilä, 1974). The half-life does not return to normal for at least two weeks after the barbiturate is discontinued. This interaction is clinically significant and may reduce the serum concentration of the standard dosage of the antibiotic to below therapeutic levels. The mechanism of this action is believed to be the induction of hepatic mircrosomal enzymes.

Griseofulvin.   Phenobarbital is reported to impair the absorption of griseofulvin (Hansten, 1972).

Monoamine Oxidase Inhibitors.   Monoamine oxidase inhibitors isocarboxazid (Marplan®), phenelzine (Nardil®), and tranylcypromine (Parnate®), which are used in the treatment of depression, prolong the effects of barbiturates, probably because metabolism of the barbiturates is inhibited. The mechanism for this action, however, is not well established (Hansten, 1972). If barbiturates are used concurrently with monamine oxidase inhibitors, reduced dosages are recommended (American Medical Association, 1973).

Tricyclic Antidepressants.   Barbiturates stimulate the metabolism of tricyclic antidepressants and therefore decrease their effectiveness (Hansten, 1972). When toxic doses of tricyclic antidepressants are taken, barbiturates may add to respiratory depression. Benzodiazepines such as diazepam (Valium®) may be the desired agents to treat the seizures produced by tricyclic antidepressant toxicity.

Phenothiazines.   Phenobarbital increases the metabolism of chlorpromazine (Thorazine®), presumably by inducing liver microsomal enzymes. The urinary excretion of conjugated chlorpromazine also increases after phenobarbital has been ingested (Hansten, 1972). These effects are observed with chronic use of both drugs. The acute effects of combining phenobarbital and chlorpromazine are additive depression of the CNS.

Antihistamines.   Antihistamines can potentiate the effects of barbiturates. When used concurrently, the dosages of both drugs should be reduced (Winter, 1948). The possible potentiation of barbiturates through concomitant use of over-the-counter antihistamines commonly contained in "cold" remedies should be kept in mind because this combination may be especially hazardous to individuals with severe lung disease and respiratory insufficiency.

Although barbiturates have been available for clinical use for 70 years, little is known about how they produce their primary effect on the CNS. Most of their adverse effects, potential for addiction, and drug interactions with other drugs were discovered during clinical usage. Much of the early chemical and clinical work with barbiturates was published in German, and most clinical articles published in the American literature did not refer to this earlier work.

Before examining the subject of barbiturate abuse and its consequences, we will present an overview of medical usage. Considerations of the abuse of prescription drugs should be viewed in light of their appropriate medical uses.

Chapter 3

MEDICAL USES OF BARBITURATES

Barbiturates have been among the drugs most commonly prescribed for the treatment of anxiety, insomnia, and convulsive disorders. Their widespread use for the treatment of anxiety and insomnia was largely unchallenged until the 1950s, when a series of new compounds, which were initially believed to be free of some of the disadvantages of barbiturates, were introduced. The first of these compounds, meprobamate, was labeled a "minor tranquilizer." Initially, drug-company advertising emphasized the fact that these compounds did not belong to the barbiturate chemical class and, by extension, implied that they were nonaddictive and would not induce physical dependency.

What evolved was a pattern of introduction of new agents and subsequent disappointment. Each drug was believed to be superior to the barbiturates and was released for clinical use. Later, reports of deaths caused by overdose would appear, followed by reports of physical dependence similar to that caused by barbiturates. Finally, a consensus would develop that the new drugs were similar to barbiturates in terms of their therapeutic spectrum, toxicity, and ability to produce physical dependence. Although these drugs could be used as alternatives for patients who were allergic to barbiturates, they were not pharmacologically advantageous for the majority of patients. The last of the compounds to be introduced was methaqualone, which is now well known for its potential for abuse.

The only compounds that are significantly more advantageous than the barbiturates are the benzodiazepines —chlordiazepoxide (Librium®), clorazepate (Tranxene®), diazepam (Valium®), oxazepam (Serax®), and clonazepam (Clonopin®). Flurazepam (Dalmane®) is marketed for the treatment of insomnia. Nitrazepam (Mogodon®), currently prescribed as an hypnotic in Great Britain and New Zealand, has an impressive safety record from the standpoint of overdose. A review of the benzodiazepines, including comparisons with barbiturates, has been published by Garattini, Mussini, and Randall (1973). Although abuse of the benzodiazepines does occur, their potential for abuse appears to be less than that of the barbiturates, meprobamate (Equanil®, Miltown®), ethchlorvynol (Placidyl®), and methyprylon (Noludar®). The dose of any benzodiazepine needed to produce physical dependence is at least five times greater than the therapeutic dose usually prescribed. Furthermore, these drugs are far safer than the barbiturates and other sedative-hypnotics from the standpoint of overdose. Individuals have survived massive overdoses of the benzodiazepines—involving 100 times the generally prescribed therapeutic dose. If death does occur, it is usually the result of combined overdoses of benzodiazepines and alcohol or other drugs.

PSYCHOTHERAPEUTIC USES

Sedatives or Tranquilizers

Depending on the context in which they are prescribed, barbiturates and other drugs that depress the CNS are called antianxiety agents, sedative-hypnotics, minor tranquilizers, hypnotics, or soporifics. The term minor tranquilizer is especially confusing because it implies a comparison with phenothiazines, butrophenones, and thioxanthenes, which are commonly referred to as major tranquilizers. Direct comparisons of major and minor tranquilizers are misleading, however, because their spectrum of clinical activity is different. The primary difference between a tranquilizer and a sedative is the degree of sedation or sleepiness each produces in relation to its antianxiety effects. In practice, however, this distinction is unclear, although there is some consensus that benzodiazepines produce greater antianxiety effects in relation to sedation (American Medical Association, 1973).

The distinction between sedative and hypnotic is based on clinical usage rather than on chemical properties. The hypnotic properties are an extension of the sedative properties along a dose-response continuum; in other words, small doses are used as sedatives and larger dosages are used as hypnotics. The terms hypnotic and soporific are interchangeable.

The superiority of the barbiturates over placebo in reducing anxiety has been demonstrated by numerous studies, which have been tabulated by Klein and Davis (1969). Barbiturates that are administered in doses large enough to reduce a patient's anxiety often diminish his mental alertness or cause drowsiness. Investigators who have differentiated sedative and antianxiety effects have found that low-income patients consider drowsiness to be a positive effect, whereas individuals whose jobs require mental alertness view this symptom as a negative side effect (e.g., Rickels, 1973).

Although the superiority of barbiturates over placebo in terms of antianxiety effects can easily be demonstrated if sufficient dosages are used, differences in the efficacy of barbiturates and nonbarbiturate sedatives are less impressive, and findings reported in the medical literature are frequently contradictory. The difficulties inherent in these studies include heterogenous patient populations as well as comparisons of dosages that are not of equal potency (Klein & Davis, 1969). Hollister (1973) has questioned the appropriateness of commonly used experimental designs for measuring the effects of antianxiety drugs. Most studies involve the use of chronic dosage regimens of a few weeks with fixed daily dosages. Hollister suggests an alternative design in which individual patients can use drugs as needed to relieve episodes of anxiety.

Pharmacological treatment of anxiety is generally effective and relatively inexpensive, but psychotherapists disagree about its long-term efficacy. Some believe that pharmacological treatment may interfere with psychotherapeutic solutions to problems (Lennard et al., 1971; Halleck, 1971), while others claim that the reduction of anxiety facilitates psychotherapeutic treatment (Klein & Davis, 1969). Wolpe (1969) described the ancillary use of barbiturates during behavior therapy.

Treatment of Insomnia

The short-, intermediate-, and, to a lesser degree, long-acting barbiturates have been widely prescribed for the treatment of insomnia. Although the clinical literature abounds with claims that the short-acting barbiturates are superior for producing sleep while the intermediate-acting compounds are more effective in maintaining sleep, controlled studies have failed to demonstrate these differential effects (e.g., Hinton, 1963; Lasagna, 1956).

The physiology of sleep and the consequent understanding of insomnia were largely unstudied until the mid-1950s, when Aserinsky and Kleitman (1953) and subsequently Dement and Kleitman (1957) demonstrated that sleep was a complex physiological process which occurred in five stages defined by EEG patterns.

Sleep disturbances occur in a variety of psychiatric syndromes as well as medical conditions. The realization that drugs affect the quality and quantity of the stage of sleep characterized by rapid eye movements (REM) began to raise questions about the efficacy of sleep induced by barbiturates, which acutely depress the quantity of REM sleep. If these compounds are taken chronically in low doses, some recovery of REM sleep occurs. At dosages in the range of 1,000 mg. per day, however, REM sleep is suppressed entirely. Dement (1960) deprived individuals of REM sleep by waking them whenever their EEG recordings indicated that they were entering the REM stage and noted that this stage was apparently necessary for sleep to be satisfying.

However, when heavy users of barbiturates were studied in a sleep laboratory, they were found to have practically no REM sleep and yet seemed to suffer no ill effects from dream deprivation (Kales et al., 1974). When barbiturates were withdrawn, however, these individuals experienced REM rebound and spent a higher than average percentage of sleep time in REM sleep. These findings may explain what clinicians have observed for years. Barbiturate users who begin using barbiturates during a period of insomnia initially find the drugs beneficial—i.e., it takes less time to fall asleep after going to bed and their total sleep time is increased. But as tolerance develops, the individual must increase the dosage to maintain the same sleep latency and total sleep time. If he tries to stop taking barbiturates abruptly, insomnia is even greater than before he began taking barbiturates, and when he does fall asleep, he is disturbed by vivid nightmares.

By using all-night EEG recordings, Evans and his associates (1968) demonstrated REM rebound in two female subjects after ingestion of as little as 200 mg. of amobarbital. During 26 consecutive nights on amobarbital, REM sleep was depressed below baseline for the first five days after the drug was initiated and then rose to or slightly above baseline. By the end of the second week, sleep latency increased as the amount of REM sleep rose. When the amobarbital was stopped, the subjects' total sleep time dropped abruptly for two nights and sleep latency increased. The interval between falling asleep and the first REM stage became shorter (less than 45 minutes), and the percentage of REM sleep increased. When Oswald and Priest (1965) gave two male subjects 400 mg. of amobarbital each night for ten nights and then 600 mg. for an additional eight nights, they found that it took five weeks to return to the baseline percentage of REM sleep. The subjects experienced nightmares for several nights after the drug was withdrawn.

This rebound of REM sleep may explain some cases of iatrogenically produced habituation to sleeping pills. The following case history illustrates the physiology of clinically disturbed sleep as well as some interesting psychodynamic features.

> A 30-year old woman (whose mother had died three years earlier) reported that her mother had been giving her Tuinal® (equal parts of amobarbital and secobarbital) whenever she had trouble sleeping, particularly when her husband was out of town. After her mother's death, the patient began taking Tuinal® every night; some from an old supply obtained by her mother and some from her physician. She used the drug primarily at night and was conscious of experiencing a "high" just before falling asleep. According to the patient, the largest amount she took per night was three

capsules, or 450 mg. As long as she took the Tuinal®, she slept well; when she tried to do without it, she trembled and experienced severe insomnia. She tried to treat her own dependency with 10 to 20 mg. of chlordiazepoxide (Librium®) at bedtime, but this was ineffective.

The patient felt guilty about her drug-taking behavior and feared she was addicted. When it was explained to her that her symptoms might be caused by the REM rebound phenomenon, she agreed to try the following treatment. She took 60 mg. of flurazepam (Dalmane®) at bedtime for one week, reduced the dosage to 45 mg. the second week, 30 mg. the third week, and 15 mg. the fourth week. The drug was discontinued in the fifth week. In addition, the patient and her husband received supportive psychotherapy, and she was encouraged to discuss her feelings about her mother's death. During a six-month follow-up visit, the patient said she had not resumed the use of sleeping pills.

Sleep laboratories have demonstrated a differential ability among different sedative-hypnotics to produce REM suppression and subsequent REM rebound. For example, chloral hydrate and flurazepam (Dalmane®) seem to produce more sedation with less REM suppression than do other sedative-hypnotics (Kales et al., 1968; Kales et al., 1969).

Sleep disturbances are also related to the physiological changes that accompany clinically significant depression. Although some depressed patients experience hypersomnia, most depressed patients spend less time sleeping than do nondepressed individuals. Furthermore, they wake up more often, have a lower arousal threshhold, experience more shifts between stages of sleep, and spend significantly less time in delta wave, or Stage IV sleep. Also, their REM sleep and REM latency are decreased.

Current clinical data indicates that tricyclic antidepressants may be the treatment of choice for sleep disturbances in depressed patients because these compounds produce nighttime sedation as well as an antidepressant effect. Initially, the sedative side effects of the tricyclic compounds are beneficial in reducing sleep latency. Later, as the antidepressant effects occur, sleep patterns tend to normalize. There is a temporal correlation between improved sleep patterns and relief from depression, barbiturates and other sedative-hypnotics that reduce REM sleep, although they offer immediate relief, may complicate the overall clinical syndrome of depression.

Narcotherapy and Diagnosis

Narcotherapy refers to the intravenous injection of drugs as an adjunct to psychotherapy. A variety of drugs, including sedatives, stimulants, and psychedelics—alone or in combination—have been used for this purpose. The barbiturates most commonly used in narcotherapy are thiopental sodium (Sodium Pentothal®) and amobarbital sodium (Sodium Amytal®), which are sometimes called "truth serum." Bleckwenn (1930) was the first to advocate the intravenous injection of Sodium Amytal® during therapy. In 1936 Horsley coined the term narcoanalysis; Grinker and Spiegel (1945) called a similar procedure narcosynthesis.

   The goal of narcotherapy is to produce an altered state of consciousness in which the patient's inhibitions are reduced and his unconscious conflicting material can be brought into consciousness. Although these productions may be useful for psychotherapeutic purposes, the material obtained is not necessarily factually accurate.

   Intravenous injections of barbiturates have also been used to distinguish between the catatonic stupor of schizophrenia and stuporous depressive states. After an injection of barbiturates, a depressed patient will usually become more stuporous or fall asleep. The catatonic schizophrenic will often experience a temporary remission, during which he may communicate rationally. These effects, however, are brief and transitory.

Weinstein and Malitz (1954) have used Amytal® narcosis to diagnose organic brain damage. When given Amytal®, brain-damaged patients deny their illness, become disoriented in terms of place, and misidentify the examiner. This phenomenon may also explain the confusion that barbiturates sometimes produce in the elderly.

OTHER MEDICAL USES

Treatment of Epilepsy

Barbiturates have the capacity to raise the seizure threshhold in epilepsy of the major motor type and decrease the frequency of seizures. Phenobarbital is commonly used for this purpose; the usual dose is 100 to 200 mg. per day, either alone or in combination with diphenylhydantoin (Dilantin®).

Because seizures are dramatic events, physicians as well as laymen generally view them as a medical emergency. This sometimes results in overtreatment of a single seizure with intravenous barbiturates. A single epileptic seizure can be managed by protecting the individual from secondary trauma to the head and allowing him to rest afterward. The risk involved in injecting barbiturates *during* a major motor seizure outweighs any possible benefit. If seizure activity recurs, intravenous doses of barbiturates, or preferably diazepam, can be administered between episodes. Of the barbiturates, phenobarbital has the greatest anticonvulsant efficacy; however, after intravenous administration, 10 to 20 minutes may be required to achieve maximum concentrations in the brain.

Anesthesia

Ultrashort-acting barbiturates, such as thiopental sodium (Sodium Pentothal®), can be injected intravenously to induce or sustain anesthesia during surgery or oral surgery, either by intermittent injection or by continuous infusion. For intermittent injections, a 2.5 per cent aqueous solution is ordinarily preferred over stronger solutions, which are more irritating to the vein. Thiopental is often injected into a freely running intravenous infusion to dilute the drug. Since barbiturates are poor analgesics, they are seldom used alone and are usually supplemented with inhalation anesthetics or with analgesics. The degree of clinical analgesia bears little relationship to the degree of cerebral depression. Doses of thiopental that are almost sufficient to produce apnea are necessary before reflex movements to painful stimuli are completely abolished.

The chief advantage of using barbiturates as anesthetics is their rapid and pleasant induction. Complications include extravenous injection; coughing; and chest-wall, laryngeal, or bronchial spasm. Bronchial spasm is most likely to occur in individuals with allergic conditions such as bronchial asthma. The only absolute contraindication to barbiturate anesthesia is in cases of acute intermittent porphyria, which is exacerbated by barbiturates and may result in death (Dean, 1953; Dundee, 1969; Dundee, McCleery & McLoughlin, 1962; Jorgenson & With, 1947). The current status of barbiturates as anesthetic agents has been reviewed by Dundee and Wyant (1974).

Antidotes to Stimulants

In 1921 Hofvendahl demonstrated that convulsions induced in animals by toxic doses of cocaine could be stopped by barbital. In addition, animals given lethal doses of cocaine survived if they had been pretreated with subcutaneous injections of barbital. Tatum, Atkinson, and Collins (1925) found that intravenous barbital or a mixture of barbital and paraldehyde could control cocaine convulsions in dogs. This antagonist effect has been used extensively during surgery under local anesthesia, especially in ear, nose, and throat surgery and in bronchoscopy. According to Wesseling (1973), diazepam can be used as an alternative.

Enzyme Inducers

Many of the drug interactions produced by barbiturates are related to the barbiturates' ability to activate drug-metabolizing enzymes in the liver. When this reduces the blood concentrations of a second drug, the activation of enzymes is considered an undesirable side effect. However, the ability of barbiturates to induce enzyme activity can be used therapeutically.

In 1966 Yaffe et al. reported that phenobarbital could be used to treat congenital nonobstructive, nonhymolytic jaundice—a disease caused by functional impairment of the glucuronyl-transference enzyme system. Because phenobarbital stimulates this enzyme system, it leads to a decrease in serum bilirubin. In 1968 Mauer and his colleagues reported that the administration of phenobarbital to pregnant women reduced the incidence of physiological jaundice in neonates. This condition is currently treated by exposing the infant to ultraviolet light after delivery.

Although barbiturates still have medical uses, they have been supplanted to a great extent by the benzodiazepines. The other "nonbarbiturate" hypnotics offer no clear therapeutic advantages in terms of efficacy or therapeutic benefits versus lethality. Phenobarbital is still the most widely used, least toxic, and most effective anticonvulsant for the treatment of major motor seizures (Drugs for epilepsy, 1976).

In November 1973 the Drug Enforcement Administration moved pentobarbital, secobarbital, and amobarbital from Schedule III to Schedule II, which placed these barbiturates under the same control as morphine and imposed restrictions on their prescription. Prescriptions for these drugs must now be written and signed by physicians who are licensed to prescribe Schedule II drugs. Prescriptions cannot be telephoned to the druggist except in an emergency; in this case, a written prescription must be supplied to the pharmacist within 72 hours. Refills are not permitted. Butabarbital and some nonbarbiturate sedative-hypnotics are in Schedule III. Phenobarbital, barbital, and the benzodiazepines are in Schedule IV.

Chapter 4

MISUSE AND ABUSE OF
BARBITURATES

Case reports of barbiturate abuse began to appear in the German literature shortly after barbital (Veronal®) was introduced into medical practice in 1903. In that year, Gerhartz reported a case of chronic intoxication, and hundreds of case studies since then have documented the fact that certain patients, when barbiturates are prescribed for them, will increase their dosage beyond the prescribed amounts. Some of these individuals will eventually develop medical or psychiatric sequelae and come to the attention of a physician.

Many heroin addicts view the barbiturates as acceptable, albeit second-choice substances for injection (Chambers, 1969; Cumberlidge, 1968; Hamburger, 1964). Supplemental use of oral barbiturates and diazepam commonly occurs among heroin addicts, including those in methadone maintenance programs. Although sporadic reports of intravenous use of barbiturates as a primary drug appeared over the years, the practice did not become widespread among youths until the development of the drug subcultures of the mid-1960s. Along with an overall increase in the use of psychoactive drugs among youths at that time, there was a dramatic increase in the use of barbiturates. Most of these young people injected barbiturates episodically but soon dropped the practice when they saw the abscesses, tissue sloughing, and deaths from overdose that were occurring. Some gave up barbiturates altogether, but the majority began taking them orally. Although young people who use barbiturates as recreational drugs have attracted the most attention, the chronic use of barbiturates in dosages beyond the prescribed therapeutic range by individuals who initially took prescribed barbiturates to alleviate insomnia or anxiety is quantitatively much greater. The National Commission on Marijuana and Drug Abuse (1973) compared the prevalence of barbiturate use to that of opiates at the turn of the century and concluded that overuse of barbiturates is America's hidden drug problem.

There is, however, some evidence that the prevalence of barbiturate use is beginning to decline. The Drug Enforcement Administration and the National Institute on Drug Abuse co-sponsor a nationwide reporting system of adverse drug experiences called Drug Abuse Warning Network (DAWN), the largest drug monitoring system in the United States. This project was designed to provide a nationwide sample of the type and extent of drug abuse occurring in 29 cities across the country. The monitored facilities include emergency rooms, crisis intervention centers, and hospitals as well as medical examiners. Figure 4.1 shows the total number of amobarbital, pentobarbital, and secobarbital mentions that appeared in the DAWN data between July 1973 and December 1974. These mentions include overdoses—suicidal and accidental—as well as medical complications of barbiturate abuse. The downward trend beginning in December 1973 does not appear to be an artifact of reporting because the number of pheno-barbital mentions continued to increase. The Domestic Council Drug Abuse Task Force (1975) estimated the total number of regular users of barbiturates who were "in trouble" to be 300,000 and noted that the unsupervised use of prescription drugs by youths has leveled off since 1972.

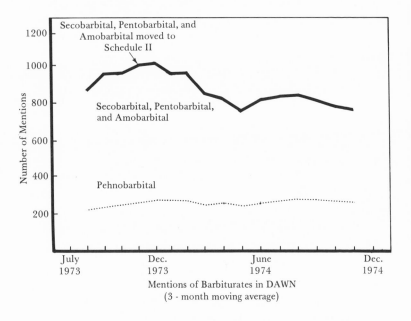

Figure 4.1   Total mentions of secobarbital, pentobarbital and amobarbital occurring in the Drug Abuse Warning Network (DAWN) between July 1973 and December 1974. (Three-month moving average)

Definition of Misuse and Abuse

Unlike the use of heroin, which is generally considered synonymous with abuse, a distinction must be made between the legitimate use of barbiturates and their misuse and abuse. As with the amphetamines, opiates, and other classes of drugs with demonstrated medical usefulness, this distinction is best considered within the context of medical uses.

The label "barbiturate abuse" is likely to be applied to individuals living on the fringes of the dominant culture rather than to those living within it who use similar amounts of barbiturates. The latter group's behavior is more likely to be labeled misuse or overuse. In other words, distinctions between abuse, misuse, and overuse of barbiturates involve a judgment that one individual makes about another's drug-taking behavior. This judgment is influenced by the user's social position, age, and occupation; the quantities of drug he takes; the reason he takes it (e.g., to obtain pleasure, reduce tension, induce sleep, commit suicide); whether he takes it orally or by injection; the source from which he obtains it (e.g., a physician, a friend, an illicit source); and the occupation and training of the person making the judgment (also see Szasz, 1974).

Parents, physicians, lawyers, judges, ministers, and teachers are likely to view barbiturate-using behavior differently. In addition to their knowledge about drugs, their judgments will be influenced by their individual life experiences; their own involvement with drugs; and their beliefs and values concerning proper medical use of barbiturates, appropriate ways of obtaining pleasure or relief from suffering, the individual's right to pursue activities that are potentially dangerous socially or medically, and the role of good government in protecting citizens from potentially dangerous activities, even when they do not want its protection. In view of this list of variables, which is by no means comprehensive, it is not surprising that there is disagreement over which barbiturate-taking behavior constitutes abuse, misuse, or overuse and which behavior should be considered legitimate or beneficial.

The common practice of equating all nonmedically supervised use of barbiturates with abuse is ineffectual and has caused much of the confusion about the severity and magnitude of barbiturate abuse. The different patterns of nonprescribed use of barbiturates range from taking another person's pills occasionally to alleviate insomnia to taking pills chronically or injecting the drug for the "rush" effect (an intensely warm, drowsy feeling that occurs immediately after the injection). Each pattern has its own attendant risks.

Because of this lack of consensus, an author who insists on using the term drug abuse should include an explicit definition. The Committee on Alcoholism and Addiction (1965) of the American Medical Association (AMA) defined barbiturate abuse as the "self-administration of excessive quantities of barbiturates leading to tolerance, physical and psychological dependence, mental confusion and other symptoms of abnormal behavior [p. 674]." Einstein and Garitano (1972), emphasizing the cultural values involved in definitions, defined abuse as "behavior, so designated by professionals and other community representatives, describing the use of particular drugs in particular ways for particular reasons which are contrary to the agreed upon rituals in a given community at a given point in time [p. 323]." Similarly, Jaffe (1975) has defined abuse as "the use, usually by self-administration, of any drug in a manner that deviates from the approved medical or social patterns within a given culture [p. 284]."

In operational terms, we define barbiturate abuse as self-prescribed use of barbiturates in a way that interferes with an individual's health or economic or social functioning. This definition separates misuse from abuse on the basis of consequences; it does not directly consider the *pattern* of use. An allergic reaction or an automobile or industrial accident following a single self-prescribed dose of barbiturates would be defined as abuse. On the other hand, chronic usage—even of amounts beyond the therapeutic range—that does not result in adverse consequences to the individual would not be defined as abuse (Wesson, Gay & Smith, 1972).

MEDICAL MISUSE

In a position statement prepared by the AMA's Committee on Alcoholism and Addiction (1965), medical misuse of barbiturates was defined as a potentially dangerous style of therapy involving sedatives. For example, the following situations were defined as misuse on the physician's part, whether or not the patient exhibited a significant degree of tolerance or physical dependence:

1. Utilizing prolonged and unsupervised administration of barbiturates for symptomatic relief, often without adequate diagnosis or knowledge of the patient's past experience with medications or attitude toward drugs.
2. Acceding to the patient's demands for increased quantities of the drug because of reported lack of symptom control accompanied by increases in nervous irritability and insomnia. These demands are often the result of developing tolerance to the effect of the drug. Neglect of periodic check-ups and family consultations may also lead to an increase in the patient's barbiturate intake beyond the proper therapeutic range for that particular patient and lead to undesirable effects.
3. Shifting from barbiturates to the newer sedatives in the mistaken belief of safety from abuse. The increasing number of patients heavily dependent on the substitute drugs attests to the danger of this practice.
4. Writing refillable prescriptions for barbiturates or their substitutes without thought of cumulative effects, additive action with other depressants, or the possible establishment of strong psychological or physical dependence. Since quantities of barbiturates well beyond the therapeu-

tic range are necessary to create physical dependence, the physician has little defense for over-prescribing. Such practices are indulged in only by physicians ignorant of, or willing to ignore, the hazards involved [p. 674].

The following case history illustrates how a physician can unwittingly contribute to drug abuse through well-intentioned but poor prescribing practices.

> A 24-year-old white male was brought into the Haight-Ashbury Free Medical Clinic in a comatose state and was treated for drug overdose using supportive measures. Subsequently, the staff discovered that the patient had taken five 100 mg. secobarbital capsules and a large quantity of alcohol. After successful resuscitation, he was hospitalized for barbiturate and alcohol detoxification.
>
> A general practitioner in the community was the patient's source of secobarbital. The patient was eligible for Medi-Cal (California's medical public assistance program), and as soon as he obtained his card each month, he went to the physician with complaints of insomnia, and once a month the physician gave him a prescription for 30 secobarbital capsules (100 mg. each) with instructions to take one capsule each night at bedtime. After filling the prescription, the patient consumed all 30 capsules, mixed with large amounts of alcohol, within three to five days. After this alcohol/barbiturate binge was over, he would visit other physicians and request additional secobarbital. He supplemented these prescriptions by purchasing additional secobarbital on the street. The first physician was unaware of the patient's barbiturate/alcohol abuse problem and had been prescribing secobarbital for his insomnia for many months.

Overuse of Prescriptions

Although physicians have been widely criticized for over-prescribing sedatives, including barbiturates, most critics have a clear antidrug bias and do not address the complex issue of the overall quality of a patient's life or his ability to function. Unwarranted use of tranquilizers is certainly not benign, but withholding sedative-hypnotics when they are indicated is also less than optimal medical practice.

Kaufman et al. (1972) designed the following comprehensive program for reducing the amount of sedative-hypnotic drugs distributed in a clinic that served 6,000 native Americans. Clinic staff, patients, and other physicians in the community were informed about the problem of sedative-hypnotic drug abuse, and brochures emphasizing the staff's willingness to discuss drug-related problems were distributed to all patients. The similarity between sedative-hypnotics and alcohol also was stressed. The clinic's social workers and pharmacists also participated actively in the care of patients with drug problems. Although most patients were willing to stop using tranquilizers after reading the brochure and talking with staff, some were angry about being deprived of their drugs. If the clinic physician was unable to manage the patient's problems, he called in a psychiatrist, social worker, or public health nurse for consultation. Kaufman and his colleagues indicated that these techniques revealed drug problems which had been masked for years. The program also yielded a 52 per cent decrease in the number of tranquilizing pills dispensed by the clinic and a 33 per cent drop in the total number of prescriptions for these drugs.

A study of the use of diazepam (Valium®) among psychiatric inpatients (Winstead et al., 1974) may be equally applicable to the use of barbiturate sedatives and perhaps to barbiturate hypnotics. As a control, Winstead and his associates wrote an order in the patients' charts for 10 mg. of diazepam (Valium®) every four hours, if needed, during the first two months of the study. Patients were not told routinely that the drug was available. After the initial two months, patients who remained on the ward or were subsequently admitted received a copy of the following statement:

> Many patients feel anxious at times during their illness. Sometimes it helps to talk to another person about what is making you feel worried or tense, and at other times it may help you to take a sedative medication.
>
> During your stay on this ward please feel free to approach any of the attendants, orderlies, nurses or doctors if you are unusually anxious, tense or worried. They will be happy to talk to you about your feelings and to give you medications if they consider it would be helpful [p. 349].

During the study, the patients had more frequent contact with nurses, received extra counseling, and were never denied diazepam when they requested it. More than one-fourth of the patients never asked for drugs, and the total number of requests from the remainder averaged one every three days.

In 1974 the AMA's Committee on Alcoholism and Drug Dependence published the following guidelines for physicians concerning prescriptions for barbiturates and barbiturate-like drugs:

1. Use barbiturates and other sedative-hypnotics for relief of severe symptoms, but avoid them for minor complaints of distress or discomfort.
2. Attempt to diagnose and treat underlying disorders before relying on drugs of this class for symptomatic relief.
3. Assess susceptibility of the patient to drug abuse before prescribing barbiturates or any other psychoactive drugs. Weigh benefits against hazards.
4. Use dosages that will not lower sensory perception, responsiveness to the environment, or alertness below safe levels.
5. Know how to administer barbiturates when clinically indicated for withdrawal in cases of drug dependence of the barbiturate type.
6. Using periodic check-ups and family consultations, monitor possible development of dependence in patients who are on an extended sedative-hypnotic regimen.

7. Prescribe no greater quantity of a drug than is needed until the next check-up.

8. Warn patients to avoid possible adverse effects because of interactions with other drugs, including alcohol.

9. Counsel patients as to the proper use of medication, e.g., follow directions on the label, dispose of old medicine no longer needed for medicinal reasons, keep medicine out of reach of children, do not "share" prescription drugs with others.

10. Convey to patients through your own attitude and manner that drugs, no matter how helpful, are only one part of an overall plan of treatment and management [p. 1441].

Behavioral Control

Barbiturates—either alone or in combination with phenothiazines—are used for behavioral control in prisons, nursing homes, and mental hospitals. Medication is given on an involuntary basis to individuals to make them more manageable, prevent complaints, and so forth. This pseudomedical use of barbiturates is not only deplorable but a perversion of the physician's role and medical ethics. There are, of course, times when a patient or inmate may become so acutely disturbed that chemical restraint may be in his own as well as the staff's best interests. But using barbiturates primarily as a convenience or to quiet inmates or patients who object to mistreatment or improper conditions is far from ethical. Obviously, barbiturates are not the only drugs that can be used in this manner.

NONMEDICAL MISUSE

Our health-oriented definition of drug abuse is the self-administration of a drug in a quantity or a pattern that impairs an individual's health or social or economic functioning. This definition implies a transitional phase between the time that a person first begins using barbiturates in a manner at variance with prescribed medical supervision and the time when his functioning is impaired.

We define this transitional phase as a period of nonmedical misuse. It includes the interval between the time an individual begins to take medication in dosages beyond those prescribed or for reasons other than medical ones and the time when drug abuse can be diagnosed. We contrast this nonmedical misuse with nonmedical *use*, which involves the self-prescription of barbiturates in dosages and patterns that approximate medical usage. For example, occasionally using a friend's secobarbital to induce sleep would not be considered misuse if the individual restricts himself to commonly prescribed therapeutic dosage because this pattern approximates generally accepted medical usage. If, however, the dosage escalates above the generally prescribed range of between 100 and 200 mg., we would label this pattern as misuse.

In the following case history, the transitional phase was easily documented because the patient saved his receipts for prescriptions for tax purposes:

> When a physician discovered that a 38-year-old male patient was using excessive amounts of Fiorinal® (a product consisting of 50 mg. of butalbital, 40 mg. of caffeine, 200 mg. of aspirin and 130 mg. of phenacetin), he refused to give the patient additional prescriptions unless the patient sought treatment for his dependence. The patient had begun using Fiorinal® tablets five years earlier to alleviate headaches that his internist had diagnosed as functional in origin. The patient claimed he had always obtained the medication by prescription, either his own or his wife's. His use of Fiorinal® was unusual in that he ground up the Fiorinal® tablets and repackaged them in 00 capsules, each of which held three tablets. If excessive sedation became a problem, he added bulk caffeine to the capsules.

This patient offered a rare opportunity to examine the progression of drug-taking behavior. Because he had receipts for his prescriptions, it was possible to plot the number of pills he took over a given interval. As indicated in Figure 4.2, the escalation phase was apparently related to the patient's conscious decision to eliminate psychic pain. Once the pattern of escalation began, it increased in a linear fashion until his internist discovered the problem and referred the patient for treatment.

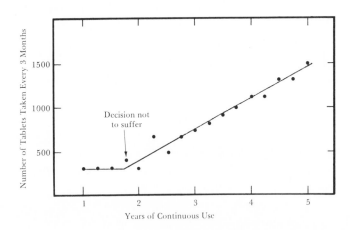

Figure 4.2 Number of Fiorinal® tablets taken by 38-year-old male patient as a function of years of use.

Multiple Drug Use

Barbiturate users are often multiple drug users, and their pattern of drug use may change over a period of time: for example, they may shift to alcohol when barbiturates are unavailable. Those who inject barbiturates intravenously take oral doses of other sedative-hypnotics, such as methaqualone (Quaalude®, Sopor®, Optimil®, Parest®, Somnafac®), or combine barbiturates with opiates, either simultaneously or sequentially, especially when the opiate of choice is in short supply.

Suicide

Barbiturates are widely known[1] to be effective suicidal agents. An accidental overdose can also occur if an individual who is intoxicated with alcohol takes barbiturates to fall asleep and thus produces an additive depressant effect. Because the labeling of intentional overdose as drug abuse is not consistently applied in the drug abuse literature, confusion occurs when studies are compared.

Antidote to Effects of Other Drugs

Barbiturates are frequently self-prescribed to counteract the irritability, paranoia and insomnia that result from intravenous use of methamphetamine, to suppress the anxiety related to LSD flashbacks, or to alleviate the symptoms of heroin withdrawal. Dependence on barbiturates may develop as a secondary pattern of drug abuse despite the fact that the barbiturate was initially used to counteract anxiety, depression, or paranoid symptoms that were secondary to the use of amphetamines or psychedelic drugs.

The usual pattern of taking high doses of intravenous methamphetamine is known as the speed cycle and can be described as an action-reaction phenomenon. The onset of the drug's effects is the action phase or high, during which the individual is hyperactive and may continue to inject methamphetamine many times a day to reexperience the rush it gives him. Because of marked stimulation, the individual is unable to sleep and does not eat as a result of the drug's anorexic effect. As progressively larger amounts of methamphetamine accumulate in his body, he may become increasingly irritable and suspicious and develop an overt paranoid psychosis. The high level of energy associated with paranoia may result in unpredictable and sometimes violent behavior.

For a variety of reasons, including fatigue, paranoia, and a dwindling supply of methamphetamine, the individual eventually stops injecting the drug and, in an effort to rest or sleep, may resort to extremely large doses of a sedative-hypnotic or opiate, as illustrated by the following case:

> A 23-year-old white male came to the Haight-Ashbury Free Medical Clinic for treatment of a gangrenous left hand. He had been injecting amphetamine in a speed run and had been unable to sleep for approximately two days. Although he had found it difficult to obtain secobarbital on the street, he had been able to obtain eight to twelve 125 mg. tablets of Doriden® (glutethimide)—a preparation he had never used before. Because of the severe anxiety, agitation, and insomnia associated with his speed run, he took all the glutethimide at once and was unconscious for two days, lying on his left hand. This was sufficient to produce pressure necrosis of his hand and necessitated the amputation of two fingers.

Heroin Substitute

When the supply of heroin is low, diluted, or too costly, heroin addicts sometimes supplement their habit with intravenous injections of short-acting barbiturates to produce a rush that is similar to the one produced by heroin. They may increase their dose of barbiturates to levels high enough to cause a combined physical dependence on barbiturates and heroin. Also, some addicts use the short-acting barbiturates to withdraw from heroin, not appreciating the fact that there is no cross-tolerance between opiates and sedative-hypnotics. As a result, we have seen a number of unintentional overdoses of barbiturates, some of which resulted in death, because individuals ingested or injected unusually large amounts of a short-acting barbiturate in the erroneous belief that a significantly high tolerance to opiates meant a similar degree of tolerance to barbiturates. In emergency rooms, mixed-drug overdose cases, particularly those resulting from a combination of opiates and sedative-hypnotics, are becoming increasingly common.

ASSESSMENT OF MOTIVATION FOR USE OF BARBITURATES

Determining a person's motivation for barbiturate use is central to developing a rational treatment plan. There are a variety of methods for determining his motivation. Most clinical assessments of and research on motivation are based on reports of abusers themselves, either through interviews or questionnaires. Experienced observers, however, frequently find discrepancies between a patient's actual behavior and the behavior that would be predicted, based on his statements concerning his motivation. This seems to be especially true among users of high doses of barbiturates, alcohol, and other drugs that impair judgment.

An analysis of the motivation for barbiturate use also may include an assessment of the user's personality structure and psychopathology and an attempt to relate these findings to his pattern of drug use. The problem with this approach is that it is difficult to establish a *causal* relationship between an individual's personality structure or psychopathology and his drug-using behavior.

A third method is to determine how and under what circumstances the individual uses drugs. His motivation is then determined by deductive reasoning. But because a person's drug-taking behavior cannot be directly observed, the data on which these deductions are based are subject to both unconscious distortion and willful deceit. Nonetheless, most individuals find it easier to describe accurately *what* they do than why they do it. Thus we favor this method for clinical purposes. Although it is assailable from several theoretical standpoints, it provides a rational basis for designing treatment intervention.

Disinhibition

The use of alcohol to produce disinhibition is socially acceptable in most segments of American society. For example, cocktail parties are designed to enhance social interaction by disinhibiting the individual's ability to critique his own behavior and thus allow a more fluid social interaction. When disinhibition is accompanied by an exaggerated elevation of mood, it is called disinhibition euphoria. Disinhibition, however, does not necessarily lead to euphoria, which depends to a large degree on a person's mental state and the environment in which his drug use occurs as well as on the drug's psychopharmacological effects. For instance, some individuals use disinhibition to express anger or resentment more freely. Disinhibition can be achieved with a wide variety of drugs and to some extent explains the fact that some individuals exhibit similar behavior while under the influence of drugs with different pharmacological effects. Some individuals who use drugs to achieve disinhibition find that stimulants and depressants are more or less interchangeable in this respect.

The following case history illustrates the use of barbiturates to achieve disinhibition:

> A 25-year-old divorced woman, the mother of a small child, voluntarily sought treatment for her dependence on barbiturates. She related that two years earlier, she had been raped by two men and subsequently had developed fears that impaired her ability to communicate with others or hold a job that required social interaction. She also developed

significant depressive symptoms, including loss of appetite and sexual drive, and sleep disturbances, which interfered with her life on a variety of levels, such as caring adequately for her child. She denied that these symptoms had existed prior to the rape.

The patient had been treated by a physician who prescribed secobarbital for her insomnia and as a daytime antianxiety agent. She discovered that if she took four secobarbital capsules (400 mg.) per day, she was able to achieve a level of disinhibition that allowed her to work and interact socially. But it soon became difficult to maintain this level of barbiturate use through legitimate prescriptions, so she tried to borrow secobarbital from friends. When they began to ask why she had to use so much, she realized that she was becoming involved in a serious "drug hustle." Furthermore, she found that without secobarbital, she drank alcohol constantly, and she became concerned about a possible drinking problem.

When the patient tried to obtain secobarbital from a hospital clinic, she was referred to the San Francisco Polydrug Project. After extensive evaluation, a treatment plan was initiated and her secobarbital usage was decreased to two capsules (200 mg.) per day. She was also given amitriptyline (Elavil®), which reduced her depressive symptoms significantly: her appetite returned, her social and sexual interactions improved, and she was able to care for her daughter satisfactorily. The patient was encouraged to begin psychotherapy with a female psychiatrist and to remain under medical supervision. Although she vigorously resisted the psychotherapist, who reminded her of her cold, dominating mother, she did accept supportive counseling from her male physician, who reminded her of her loving and supportive father. Attempts to reduce the patient's secobarbital intake to less than 200 mg. per day resulted in an increased intake of alcohol to achieve a level of social disinhibition comparable to that reached with 200 mg. or more of secobarbital.

The use of drugs as disinhibitory agents does not necessarily lead to addiction, nor is it always maladaptive. Many social gatherings are improved by the moderate use of alcohol. Some individuals are able to capitalize on their life experiences in a mildly disinhibited state and transfer their behavior to the drug-free state. This technique has been used therapeutically to desensitize phobic patients by giving them tranquilizers and asking them to face the situation that elicits the phobic reaction (Wolpe, 1969).

There is usually an upper limit to the degree of drug-induced disinhibition that can be transferred to the drug-free state. For example, individuals who become more than mildly disinhibited may find that the experience can only be reproduced when they are intoxicated with drugs. This phenomenon, called state-dependent learning, has been studied extensively in animals and may explain why some individuals seem unable to transfer the behavior they learned in an intoxicated state to the nonintoxicated state. To duplicate the behavior, the individuals must continue their use of drugs and consequently become psychologically dependent on them.

Self-exploration and Self-medication of Psychopathology

Individuals often claim that they take psychedelics, stimulants, and marijuana to bypass psychic defenses, provide greater access to the unconscious, facilitate understanding of self, or obtain insight into a personal problem. We have never encountered an individual who convinced us that he took barbiturates for this purpose, although some barbiturates, particularly sodium amobarbital, are administered medically to recover repressed memories.

The relationship between psychiatric symptomatology and use of barbiturates has been the subject of much speculation. Some individuals apparently continue to take self-prescribed barbiturates because the drugs are partially effective in decreasing dysphoria or auditory hallucinations. The coexistence of depression and barbiturate use does not necessarily establish that a person is using barbiturates to alleviate a dysphoric mood. More evidence is needed to determine his motivation. For example, he may state that "I only use drugs when I'm down and trying to get up." Although this type of statement does not establish absolute causality, it does lend credence to a link between dysphoric mood and drug use. This assessment can be quite difficult to make, however. First, the dysphoric state may be the result of previous drug use or may occur spontaneously without drug use. Second, the user's vocabularly may make it difficult to distinguish between self-medication of anxiety or dysphoria and pleasure-seeking. And third, drug users may use the same drug for different reasons. The key to sorting out these confusing issues is to obtain a detailed history of the circumstances in which drug use occurs. If a patient consistently uses drugs when in a dysphoric mood and if he seems chronically depressed, the implications for treatment are quite different than they would be for a patient who uses stimulants episodically to achieve euphoria.

When working with depressed patients, it is important to determine whether their depression is episodic or alternates with periods of elation and whether there is a relationship between their drug use and depressive episodes. Patients who have recurrent fluctuations in mood often benefit from lithium maintenance; so does an occasional patient who exhibits unipolar cyclical depressive episodes alone. Tricyclic antidepressants such as imipramine (Presamine®, Tofranil®) or amitriptyline (Elavil®) are also worth a therapeutic trial when treating chronically depressed individuals. Because lithium and tricyclic antidepressants can be toxic, they must be monitored closely. An adequate trial with tricyclic antidepressants consists of dosages of 150 mg. or more per day for at least one month. With lithium therapy, blood levels must be monitored to assess therapeutic levels. The dosages may vary from 600 to 1,800 mg. per day to achieve therapeutic blood levels (0.5 to 1.5 meg/1) in different individuals.

The relationship between psychotic symptomatology (e.g., hallucinations) and drug use is generally easier to assess than is depression. Statements such as "I use the barbiturates to quiet the voices" are fairly convincing unless the psychotic symptomatology itself is caused by withdrawal from sedative-hypnotics or alcohol. The relation between medical illness and drug use has also created considerable controversy. As with psychopathology, demonstration of medical illness in a drug user does not necessarily establish a cause-and-effect relationship. In our experience, pain from almost any source, including trauma, can be instrumental in the development of addiction, especially to opiates and opioids but also to sedatives.

Facilitation of Performance

The use of stimulants to facilitate psychic or motor performance is well known, as evidenced by publicity about the widespread use of stimulants among professional athletes. It is not as well known that barbiturates are used to facilitate performance. On a pharmacological basis, one would predict that barbiturates would decrease motor coordination (and this indeed occurs at intoxicating dosages), but at subintoxicating doses, coordination can actually be enhanced. This phenomenon probably occurs indirectly as disinhibition develops and self-consciousness decreases. With practice, one can learn to overcome any initial mild motor impairment that may occur. We have observed individuals playing pool or a musical instrument whose motor performance appeared to be facilitated by barbiturates: i.e., they performed better after taking the drug in subintoxicating amounts. A musician seen at the San Francisco Polydrug Project found that the disinhibiting and anxiety-reducing properties of secobarbital were essential to his performance and took two secobarbitals before each musical set. This behavior may be related to state-dependent learning.

Barbiturates can also affect sexual performance markedly. For example, we have treated men whose initial motivation for taking barbiturates was self-medication of premature ejaculation and women who used barbiturates to reduce their sexual inhibitions so they could experience orgasm.

Escape

Social theorists are prone to relating all drug-using behavior to adverse social conditions such as poverty and racism: i.e., they view drug use as an escape from intolerable social situations. Although this theory is perhaps applicable to those who live in depressed socioeconomic environments, it cannot be applied to persons from more privileged socioeconomic backgrounds. Drug use in the latter population is more likely to be motivated by the desire to escape internal states such as boredom, loneliness, and other intrapsychic distress.

Because of the wide variety of motivations for using barbiturates, it is not surprising that descriptions of patterns of use focus only on which drug is used or on how much is used and how often. Although statistically valid, these data are not of great value when applied to individuals. Treatment plans are usually more effective when this type of data is combined with a specific individual's motivation for use.

Chapter 5

COMPLICATIONS OF BARBITURATE ABUSE

CHRONIC AND EPISODIC INTOXICATION

Some persons tend to overuse any drug that will lessen their anxiety or induce a state of mild disinhibition. Furthermore, they are likely to be introduced to barbiturates by physicians, who prescribed the drugs as mild tranquilizers or sleeping pills. Many of these individuals do not identify with the drug-using subculture; they simply find that barbiturates make it easier to cope with life. As their tolerance to the drug's tranquilizing and sedative effects develops, they increase the dosage, often without the physician's knowledge. It is this tendency to escalate dosages against medical advice that distinguishes these individuals from others who use sedatives successfully to combat incapacitating anxiety or stress.

As these individuals increase their daily dosage, they usually begin contacting other physicians and request barbiturates for sleep problems or nervousness. Often several physicians will be prescribing drugs for these patients simultaneously, and all of them may be unaware that the patient is abusing the barbiturates he has prescribed. Frequently, these individuals remain unidentified until their confusion, irritability, inability to work effectively, and episodes of acute intoxication finally draw attention to their drug use. By this time, the degree of physical dependence may be marked. (These cases often involve a history of alcohol misuse in conjunction with the misuse of sedatives.)

> A 26-year-old beautician found that two secobarbital capsules (200 mg.) "assisted" her to function in public because of their disinhibitory and antianxiety effects. However, she also liked the drug's euphoric effects and gradually increased the dosage to between 400 and 500 mg. a day. At that level, she experienced some confusion and clouding of consciousness, her motor performance was impaired, and she was unable to work effectively. As a result, her employer fired her.

The pattern of episodic intoxication is found most commonly among teen-agers and young adults, who take enough barbiturates (100 to 300 mg.) orally to produce intoxication—for much the same reason that others use alcohol. Some of these young people either find alcohol distasteful or are unable to tolerate the gastric irritation it can produce. The majority, however, alternate between barbiturates and alcohol or ingest both simultaneously. Young people have told us that after ingesting secobarbital to achieve intoxication in a social setting, they were stopped by the police while driving because their motor performance was impaired. But because the breathilizer test for alcohol was negative, they could not be arrested for drunken driving.

The sources of supply for episodic users are the black market, the family medicine cabinet, and, occasionally, prescriptions. The main difficulties associated with this pattern of barbiturate use, especially in combination with alcohol, are accidental overdose, escalating involvement with drugs of many pharmacological varieties, and the dangers that are inherent in teen-age alcohol intoxication—lack of coordination, irrational behavior, and automobile accidents.

INTRAVENOUS USE

The contents of pentobarbital or secobarbital capsules can be dissolved in water and injected. The primary reason for taking the drugs this way is the rush that occurs immediately after injection. (A rush is not experienced after oral ingestion.) This pattern is usually observed in young adults who are strongly committed to the drug-using subculture.

Although this pattern of barbiturate usage probably involves a relatively small number of individuals in comparison with the other patterns described, it is by far the most hazardous. The individual rapidly develops a tolerance to the drug's intoxicating qualities and subsequently increases the dose. Tolerance to fatal doses, however, does not increase to the same degree as tolerance to intoxicating doses. Because of the rapid onset of effect, the intravenous user is far more likely than the oral user to overdose accidentally and thus runs a far greater risk of respiratory arrest and death.

Individuals who self-administer barbiturates intravenously are known as "barb freaks" and occupy a low status within the drug-using subculture. They may become so engrossed in the drug that they neglect basic hygiene and nutrition, and the lassitude produced by the drug intensifies this pattern of personal neglect.

Barbiturates are often used in conjunction with stimulants ("uppers"). Intravenous amphetamine users ("speed freaks") often resort to barbiturates to come down after prolonged abuse of amphetamines (or a "speed run"). Another variation on this pattern of barbiturate abuse involves the heroin addict who supplements his heroin with barbiturates when the supply of heroin is low or unknowingly uses barbiturates because the dealer adulturates the heroin with barbiturates. Some patients on methadone maintenance inject barbiturates after they are stabilized on methadone; the ritual surrounding the use of needles probably contributes to this behavior (Howard & Borges, 1971).

Many severe medical complications occur as a consequence of intravenous barbiturate use. The most common ones, such as cellulitis and vascular complications, make the intravenous user highly visible in free clinics, emergency rooms, and physician's offices.

Cellulitis. Solutions of barbiturates are irritating to body tissues. Cellulitis, with or without infection, occurs when barbiturates are accidentally injected subcutaneously. The tissue becomes inflamed, painful, and swollen. Unless infection develops, treatment is symptomatic; hot soaks, analgesics, and limitation of movement are helpful. A broad-spectrum antibiotic should be given if fever develops, and incision and drainage may be necessary if a definite abscess forms.

Vascular Complications. If accidentally injected into an artery, solutions of barbiturates are more likely to produce vascular complications than are heroin solutions. Users run the risk of losing a hand or fingers if they inject the drug into an artery instead of a vein. This can occur both with dissolved pills and with barbiturates that are pharmaceutically prepared for injection (Cohen, 1948). The mechanism for these vascular complications has been the subject of several theories (see Brown, Lyons & Dundee, 1968), including arterial spasm, damage to the arterial wall and thrombosis, and noradrenalin release and subsequent arterial blockage by microemboli of barbiturate cyrstals. Biopsy of affected tissue reveals thrombosis of the blood vessels.

Brown and his colleagues (1968) found that a 5 per cent solution of thiopentone, when mixed with blood in concentrations that were similar to those achieved during clinical administration into the brachial artery, invariably resulted in the formation of crystals, hemolysis of red blood cells, and platelet aggregation—any of which could produce some degree of vascular clotting. In addition, they indicated that other mechanisms of action might be involved.

The most common sites for intra-arterial injection are the flexor surface of the elbow and the wrist, where the veins and arteries lie close together. Arterial injection usually produces intense pain beyond the site of injection. In many cases the pain is severe enough to make the individual interrupt the injection. If he has applied a tight tourniquet on the extremity, however, he may not notice the pain until the tourniquet is released. Swelling, purplish discoloration, and coldness of the extremity begin soon after the injection, and the individual usually seeks treatment because of the intense pain, which can be elicited by any active or passive motion of the hands or fingers or a light touch to the skin. The fingers and hands are cyanotic and mottled along the wrist artery, or along the forearm if the brachial artery has been injected.

Because the complications associated with intra-arterial barbiturate injection constitute a medical emergency and involve complex, long-term treatment, they should be dealt with in a hospital. Gaspar and Hare (1972), surgeons at the University of Southern California School of Medicine, recommend the following treatment: (1) meperidine (Demerol®) in large amounts for five or six days to control pain, (2) elevation of the affected extremity by an overhead support made from a stockinet bandage, (3) intravenous injections of heparin sodium (10,000 units) every six hours for 24 hours, followed by 5,000 units intramuscularly every six hours for four to five days, (4) 500 ml. of low-molecular-weight dextran daily for four days to prevent sludging and thrombosis in small blood vessels, (5) 40 mg. of Decadron® (dexamethasone) every six hours for seven days to reduce edema, (6) routine doses of antacids, and (7) initiation of physiotherapy, consisting of active and passive motions and whirlpool baths, as soon as the patient can tolerate it. Gaspar and Hare do not advocate the use of antibiotics unless there is definite evidence of infection. Nor do they suggest the use of intra-arterial drugs, arteriograms, or fasciotomies.

Sometimes the symptoms of vascular insufficiency that follow the injection of barbiturates into an artery are less dramatic. The following case history, based on a malpractice case, illustrates some of the medicolegal complications that may arise:

> The 20-year-old plaintiff injected two "reds" (secobarbital) into the medial aspect of his leg (he later denied feeling pain at the time). The next day he experienced some pain and noticed that his toes felt cold to the touch. When the plaintiff went to the county hospital, a physician in the emergency room informed him that he would not be given any drugs because he had already taken enough. The physician then sent him home with instructions to cut his toenails.
>
> The second day, the plaintiff returned to the emergency room accompanied by his mother and was examined by a number of physicians, who seemed to be taking the situation lightly. For example, one physician asked "What were you trying to do, inject a vein?" and then laughed, saying "You goofed and got it into an artery." The plaintiff was sent home without treatment and told to see another doctor in about a week.
>
> On the third day, the plaintiff went to a private physician but misrepresented his history, stating that he had kicked something with his foot. The physician treated him with antibiotics, presumably because there was swelling and fever. On the fourth day, the plaintiff returned and admitted to the physician that he had injected something into his foot.

The physician then referred him to a private surgeon, who refused to accept him as a patient because he had no insurance and was not receiving public assistance. Instead, the surgeon referred him back to the county hospital's emergency room and gave him a note to show the physicians there. By the time the plaintiff was admitted to the hospital, his foot was gangrenous and was subsequently amputated. A malpractice suit was lodged against the hospital, and the case was settled out of court.

Other Medical Complications. In addition to the complications that are specific for barbiturates, the intravenous barbiturate user is also exposed to the dangers inherent in any nonmedical use of hypodermic needles: (1) serum hepatitis, (2) bacterial infections such as endocarditis, pneumonia, and tetanus, (3) syphilis and malaria, and (4) allergic reactions to adulterants that may have been added to the drug.

LETHALITY

Although the barbiturates are relatively safe when used in therapeutic dosages, 10 to 15 times the daily therapeutic dose is lethal to an individual who has not acquired tolerance for the drug. This same ratio holds for other sedative-hypnotics, with the exception of the benzodiazepines, which have a much larger margin of safety than do the barbiturates. (Individuals have taken 100 times the therapeutic dosages of the benzodiazepines and survived.)

More than 15,000 deaths secondary to barbiturate poisoning are reported each year in the United States. Without question, a high percentage of these deaths were deliberate suicides. Exact figures are impossible to obtain, however, because it is often difficult to differentiate between accidental death and suicide. Nevertheless, it is reasonable to assume that a significant percentage of these deaths are caused by accidental ingestion of barbiturates, particularly in the case of children.

These data lead some physicians, including ourselves, to believe that the benzodiazepines should be the drug of choice among hypnotic agents. Since most studies indicate that benzodiazepines and barbiturates are equally effective as hypnotic agents, the safety factor alone would dictate a preference for the benzodiazepines over barbiturates. Although we have seen patients who claim that the barbiturates are superior hypnotic agents and we acknowledge the possibility that this may in fact be true for some individuals, there is a strong possibility that their preference for barbiturates is based on the disinhibition euphoria they experience or on some idiosyncracy. Controlled studies indicate that when used chronically, the barbiturates may *not* be effective hypnotics (e.g., Kales et al., 1974). We advocate trying sedating (5-20mg.) benzodiazepines, diazepam (5-20mg.), or flurazepam hydrochloride (15-30mg.), first, especially when the patient has not developed a strong preference for a barbiturate hypnotic.

There are two pragmatic difficulties with the above suggestions, both of which involve economic factors. First, the cost per dose of benzodiazepines are generally eight to ten times that of the barbiturates. An exception is chlordiazepoxide, which is now available in generic form. Second, many public medical assistance programs (e.g., Medi-Cal in California) include barbiturates on their lists of allowed drugs but will not pay for benzodiazepine hypnotics.

In the long run, this shortsightedness may be extremely costly. Keeping one overdose patient in the intensive care unit for several days costs as much as the difference between thousands of prescribed doses of barbiturates and benzodiazepines. If one accepts our premise that the barbiturates are generally as efficacious as the benzodiazepines in terms of hypnotic action but are far more dangerous from the standpoint of overdose, one would conclude that the benzodiazepines are the superior choice. By extension, then, public medical assistance programs that force a physician to prescribe a medically inferior drug are perpetuating a double standard of treatment that favors the rich over the poor.

OVERDOSE

Because barbiturates and other sedative-hypnotic drugs are potent depressants of the central nervous system and are so easily obtained, life-threatening overdoses—both accidental and intentional—frequently occur. Intentional overdoses often involve a combination of multiple drugs and household poisons, and treatment usually must begin before the specific drug or agent has been confirmed. Table 5.1 lists several classes of common drugs that can cause coma and convulsions when taken in excessive quantities.

Differential diagnosis should include hypoglycemia, head trauma, cerebrovascular accidents, postictal (convulsive) states, and diabetic coma. Some emergency room physicians routinely administer 50 per cent glucose solution (to rule out hypoglycemia) and one cc. of Narcan® (naloxone) intravenously to rule out narcotic overdose in any patient who is comatose when admitted.

Symptoms

Patients who have taken an overdose of barbiturates or other sedative-hypnotics present a variety of signs and symptoms that must be interpreted quickly and accurately. A patient may come for treatment shortly after taking an overdose and lapse into coma later. Signs and symptoms will vary, depending on the drug or drugs ingested, the time that has elapsed since ingestion, the amount of drugs

Table 5.1 Common Drugs That in Instances of Overdose
May Cause Coma and Convulsions

Type of drug	Generic name	Brand name
Sedative-hypnotics	Methaqualone	Optimil
		Parest
		Quaalude
		Somnafac
		Sopor
Tricyclic antidepressants	(Amitriptyline &	Elavil
	perphenazine)	Etrafon
	Desipramine	Norpramin
		Pertofrane
	Doxepin	Adapin
		Sinequan
	Imipramine	Presamine
		Tofranil
	Nortriptyline	Aventyl
Antipsychotics		
Butyrophenones	Haloperidol	Haldol
Phenothiazines	Chlorpromazine	Thorazine
	Prochlorperazine	Compazine
	Trifluoperazine	Stelazine
Thioxanthenes	Chlorprothixene	Taractan
Stimulants	Amphetamine[a]	
	Dextroamphetamine[a]	
	Methamphetamine[a]	
	Street cocaine[b]	

[a]Most commonly used as the generic product.
[b]The cocaine obtained on the street is often a mixture of methamphetamine and local anesthetics: i.e., it does not contain cocaine.

ingested, the method by which they were taken (i.e., orally or intravenously), and on medical complications such as diabetes, hepatitis, asthma, heart disease, or traumatic injury, particularly to the head. Unfortunately, no specific reversal agent, such as naloxone (Narcan®), which is effective in cases of opiate overdose, is available to counteract the effects of an overdose of sedative-hypnotics.

The signs and symptoms of an overdose of sedative-hypnotics generally include slurred speech, staggering gait, sustained nystagmus, slowed reactions, lethargy, and progressive respiratory depression characterized by shallow and irregular breathing leading to coma and possibly death. Pinpoint pupils, although usually indicating opiate intoxication, do not rule out the possibility of simultaneous ingestion of opiates and sedative-hypnotics. Similarly, dilated, fixed pupils in a comatose patient do *not* rule out the possibility of opiates and may be the result of hypoxia or a combination of drugs.

When admitted, the patient may be slightly intoxicated, semiconscious, or comatose. Therefore, his history must be taken quickly to discover what drug or combination of drugs (including alcohol) and how much has been taken, when and how it was ingested, and whether any medical complications (drug or non-drug-related) are present that may aggravate the effects of the overdose. Examination of pill bottles brought in by the patient or his companions may be helpful, not only to determine what drugs are involved in the overdose but also to alert the physician to concurrent medical problems for which the patient is under treatment. In addition the prescription bottles give names of prescribing physicians and dispensing pharmacies. Anyone who accompanies the patient should be questioned. If the patient vomits, special care should be devoted to making certain that he does not aspirate the vomit, and samples of the vomit should be saved for toxicological analysis.

First Aid Management

Keeping the patient awake and moving to reduce the chances of his becoming comatose; giving him activated charcoal to delay gastric absorption; and applying general supportive measures, such as clearing an airway, maintaining respiration, keeping him warm and elevating his feet are of primary importance until he can be moved to a hospital for more definitive treatment. We strongly discourage any additional first aid measures. Stimulants should *not* be used to counteract the depressive effects of sedative-hypnotics because their side effects create additional hazards. Patients who have taken a serious overdose of sedative-hypnotics can be saved if they reach a hospital with a heartbeat and are not grossly hypoxic.

Emergency Treatment

Overdose patients can be awake, semicomatose, or comatose when they reach the emergency room. Figure 5.1 indicates the appropriate treatment plan for each stage. The principal sign that differentiates these stages is the degree of CNS depression.

Awake Patient. The patient's respiration, blood pressure, and pulse rate are evaluated, his pupils are checked, a heart and lung examination is performed, and bowel sounds are evaluated. Pertinent information is obtained from the patient, if possible, or from the persons who brought him in to determine what intoxicants he has ingested. Unfortunately, even when a friend accompanies a patient, the drug history obtained may be unreliable. Therefore, if feasible, the material the patient has ingested should be subjected to toxicological analysis as quickly as possible. If the patient is awake after the history and physical workup are completed, vomiting should be induced with syrup of ipecac rather than lavage. Lavage with a large tube is extremely difficult when the patient is semicomatose or awake. Furthermore, it is important to induce vomiting, not only to eliminate any psychoactive drug still remaining in the stomach, but to obtain a toxicological analysis of the stomach's contents.

Vomiting is also preferable to lavage in an awake patient because the first part of the small bowel is also emptied, whereas gastric lavage clears only the stomach's contents. After vomiting has been induced, the patient's

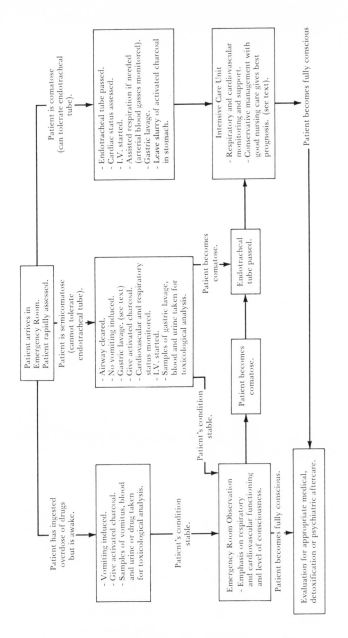

Figure 5.1 Acute treatment for overdose of barbiturates or other sedative hypnotics.

vital signs and mental status are checked every 15 minutes to determine whether he is becoming stuporous or comatose. If, after a few hours, it is apparent that CNS depression is not progressing, the patient is released to appropriate medical, detoxification, or psychiatric aftercare facilities.

Semicomatose Patient.   If the patient is semicomatose an endotracheal tube cannot be inserted to protect the airway. Vomiting should *not* be induced because he is likely to aspirate the stomach's contents. With the patient in a semirecumbent position, careful gastric lavage with 10 to 15 liters of lavage fluid is indicated if it can be determined that the drug was ingested within four hours of treatment. A slurry of activated charcoal can be instilled into the stomach through the lavage tube and be left in the stomach to retard the absorption of any material that is not removed by lavage.

The advantage of removing the unabsorbed drug from the stomach must be weighed against the danger of pulmonary aspiration that may occur during lavage. Some physicians believe that in a medical setting where prompt treatment of respiratory insufficiency can be instituted, the danger of lavage with attendant risk of aspiration is greater than the danger of progressive respiratory insufficiency and therefore do not lavage unless the patient can tolerate an endotracheal tube.

An evaluation of arterial blood gasses can be used to determine the degree of respiratory insufficiency. EKG and respiration should be monitored continuously until the patient regains consciousness and is mentally alert. He should then be released to appropriate medical, detoxification, or psychiatric aftercare facilities.

Comatose Patient.   When a patient comes into the emergency room after ingesting barbiturates or other sedative-hypnotics and is comatose (i.e., he will tolerate an endotracheal tube), a life-threatening emergency is present, and the following steps should be taken as quickly as possible:

1. Clear the airway.

2. Establish an intravenous fluid system to maintain the cardiovascular system and administer drugs rapidly.

3. Obtain a brief history and physical examination.

4. Take the vital signs.

5. Insert an endotracheal tube to guard the airway.[1]

6. Perform gastric lavage with fluid containing activated charcoal to remove any remaining psychoactive drug from the stomach and obtain material for toxicological analysis.

After these procedures have been completed, arterial blood should be drawn and analyzed for blood gasses to evaluate the degree of respiratory sufficiency. Two major prognostic signs of approaching respiratory failure and cardiovascular collapse are respiratory acidosis (the result of depressed ventilation with retained CO_2) and low blood pressure. After the patient has received emergency treatment, he should be transferred to the intensive care unit (ICU), which will continue to provide the following: respirator assisted ventilation, intravenous fluids, cardiovascular monitoring, careful monitoring of urinary output, and intensive nursing care.

The importance of the ICU nurse cannot be overemphasized. It is the nurse's skill in maintaining the airway and recognizing the early signs of decompensation that often saves a patient's life. If the ICU is not routinely involved in treating crises related to sedative-hypnotics, its nursing staff must receive special training. Clinical experience demonstrates that recovery rates are directly related to the ICU staff's degree of specialization and training in the management of specific medical problems.

Table 5.2 contains a method of estimating the degree of intoxication in patients seen in the emergency room. Sometimes called the Reed system (Reed, Driggs & Foote, 1952), this classification has been used extensively by

Table 5.2   A Classification System for Estimating the
Severity of Barbiturate Overdose

Degree of intoxication	Signs and symptoms
Group 0	Patient is asleep but can be roused and will answer, sit up in bed, drink fluids, and so on.
Group I	Patient is comatose but will withdraw from painful stimuli such as venipuncture, slapping, and pinching. There is no circulatory embarrassment and all reflexes are intact.
Group II	Patient does not withdraw from painful stimuli but has no respiratory or circulatory depression. Most or all of his reflexes are intact.
Group III	Patient's reflexes are virtually absent, but his respiration and circulation are not depressed.
Group IV	Patient's reflexes are absent, and he has respiratory depression with cyanosis, circulatory failure and shock, or both.

Source: Reed, Driggs, and Foote, 1952, pp. 290-291.

clinicians. Reed and his associates point out that a patient should not be classified until an adequate airway has been established because cyanosis and areflexia can be secondary to anoxia from obstruction of the airway. When oxygenation is reestablished, the patient can be classified in a less toxic group than seemed warranted at first.

After emergency treatment of the comatose patient has been completed, some physicians initiate measures to increase the excretion of barbiturates through forced diuresis, hemodialysis, or peritoneal dialysis. Alkalinization of the urine can be used to increase excretion of phenobarbital. These procedures, however, are not without risk and have their own rate of morbidity.

The conservative methods presented here have produced excellent results. The key to conservative management of the sedative-hypnotic overdose is skilled nursing care with constant attention to the clearing of bronchial secretions and to hypotension and cardiac arrhythmias.

Barbiturate overdose is a frequent event in medical emergency rooms. Quantitatively, the most common cause of overdose is a suicide attempt. Although overdose is generally viewed in terms of its more dramatic, acute consequences, chronic morbidity such as tissue necrosis and brain damage may produce long-term disability.

Additional Considerations

Aftercare. As mentioned earlier, when the patient is conscious, he should be transferred to medical, detoxification, or psychiatric aftercare facilities. We cannot overemphasize the importance of aftercare treatment. We have observed many cases of patients who were released without psychiatric evaluation and overdosed again within a few days, sometimes with a fatal outcome. This aspect of drug abuse treatment will be discussed more thoroughly in Chapter 7.

Mixed-drug Overdose. Increasing numbers of individuals are simultaneously using different classes of drugs. Methadone-maintenance clients, for example, take barbiturates or other sedative-hypnotics in addition to methadone.

There is no cross tolerance between sedative-hypnotics and narcotics (including methadone). If sedative-hypnotic overdose is suspected in an individual who is dependent on opiates or is being maintained on methadone, we recommend the use of the narcotic antagonist naloxone (Narcan®) to counteract any respiratory depression that may be caused by the methadone or other opiate. The response to naloxone can be helpful in determining whether methadone or another opiate is contributing to the patient's respiratory depression.

Tissue Necrosis. The anesthesia caused by a massive overdose of barbiturates may result in extensive pressure tissue necrosis, as illustrated in the following example:

In a 27-year-old male who was seen because of multiple drug abuse, an area of sloughed tissue approximately 15 centimeters in diameter was noted in the mid-sacral area. Although the wound was well healed at the time of the examination, it was obvious that skin grafts had been required to close the wound, which extended to the sacrum. The patient related that during a suicide attempt five years earlier, he had taken a large quantity of secobarbital pills—he was not certain about the exact number. Two days later, he woke up with symptoms of gangrene over the sacral area. He then went to a hospital, where extensive debridement and skin grafting were performed.

NOTES

1. Insertion of an endotracheal tube to guard the airway—both to keep it patent and to prevent aspiration of stomach contents—is a medical procedure that must be performed by an experienced anesthesiologist, surgeon, or internist. Anesthesiologists, who are often available during such emergencies, are generally the most skilled.

Chapter 6

PHYSICAL DEPENDENCY

In 1905 Kress reported a case of withdrawal seizures associated with chronic barbiturate abuse only two years after Veronal was introduced into clinical medicine. Seven years later, Laehr (1912) reported a case of psychosis caused by barbiturate withdrawal.

Until the mid-1930s, the English literature was contradictory concerning the ability of barbiturates to produce a withdrawal syndrome. Seevers and Tatum (1931), working with barbital in dogs, observed that motor unrest, ataxic movements, and convulsions occurred 48 hours after the final dose of barbital. Stanton (1936) and Swanson, Weaver, and Chen (1937) found that laboratory animals failed to demonstrate signs of withdrawal. Curran (1938) believed that convulsions in chronic users of barbiturates were caused by overdose rather than withdrawal. Tatum (1939) maintained that unlike morphine or heroin, the barbiturates did not produce "true addiction" and that the mental disturbances which characterize barbiturate withdrawal were the result of intoxication.

The issue of withdrawal was eventually clarified in the English literature by clinicians who used barbiturates for continuous sleep therapy. Although Palmer and Paine (1932) reported that their patients did not exhibit withdrawal phenomena, Palmer and Braceland (1937) observed signs and symptoms in their patients that they attributed to withdrawal. In 1942 Kalinowsky published a study of seven nonepileptic patients at Pilgrim State Hospital in Brentwood- New York, who experienced seizures four to five days after barbital was discontinued. Alexander (1951) described severe withdrawal phenomena in patients after the cessation of ten days of continuous narcosis with Sodium Amytal® (amobarbital). Although he clearly recognized that some researchers considered the withdrawal syndrome to be a *complication* of continuous narcosis, he believed that the delirium was therapeutically beneficial and attempted to produce it.

The medical aspects of barbiturate withdrawal were summarized in an excellent monograph by Wulff (1959), who not only provided a comprehensive review but made many useful clinical observations of his own patients.

WITHDRAWAL SYNDROME

The barbiturate withdrawal syndrome can be conceptualized as a spectrum of signs and symptoms that occur after barbiturate intake is stopped. With pentobarbital and secobarbital, the signs and symptoms of withdrawal begin 12 to 24 hours after the final dose, become most severe after 24 to 72 hours, and then gradually subside. The syndrome is similar for all barbiturates and sedative-hypnotics; however, with phenobarbital or barbital the onset of symptoms may not occur until 48 to 72 hours after the final dose. The signs and symptoms do not necessarily follow a specific sequence but can include anxiety, tremors, nightmares, inability to sleep, anorexia, nausea, postural hypotension, seizures, delirium, and hyperpyrexia. The severity of withdrawal is a function of the pattern of drug use, individual susceptibility, the interval between doses, and the duration of use.

During the first one to five days of untreated withdrawal, the EEG may show paroxysmal bursts of the high-voltage, slow-frequency waves that usually precede seizures. The delirium may include disorientation to time, place, and situation as well as visual and auditory hallucinations, and it is usually preceded by a period of insomnia lasting from 24 to 48 hours. Some individuals exhibit delirium alone, others experience convulsions alone, and some may manifest both delirium and convulsions.

Although the number of cases reported in the literature is small, withdrawal from high doses of barbiturates or other sedative-hypnotics such as meprobamate, if improperly treated, may cause death (Fraser et al., 1952; Meyer, 1939; Wulff, 1959; Swanson & Okada, 1963). Because the withdrawal syndrome mimics a fulminating infection, in the absence of a history of barbiturate abuse it may go undiagnosed.

One psychiatrist's failure to diagnose and treat physical dependence upon barbiturates adequately resulted in a malpractice suit:

> When a patient with a history of mental illness was admitted to a New York State mental hospital, she told the admitting physician that she was taking Nembutal® and had suffered a convulsion four years earlier and another two months before admission. The physician diagnosed her as a schizophrenic, schizoaffective type, and treated her with Thorazine® and Stelazine®. The day after admission, the patient had a seizure, a second one later, and died on the fourth day. Her

husband brought action against the state to recover damages for wrongful death and conscious pain and suffering, allegedly caused by the admitting physician's negligence and malpractice. The court held that the physician lacked the skill of the average physician in the locality to treat barbiturate addiction. With regard to diagnosis, the court held that neglecting to pursue the possibility of barbiturate addiction in the face of ample evidence was negligence and brought a judgment against the physician and the hospital. The award, however, was limited to nominal damages amounting to $5945.20 (*O'Neil* v. *State of New York*, 1971; see also, American Medical Association, 1971).

TREATMENT STRATEGIES

The majority of patients who come to a hospital emergency room with an overdose of barbiturates (or other sedative-hypnotics) are acutely intoxicated or in coma following the ingestion of a single large dose of the drug; they are not physically dependent on it. Unless the drug has been used daily for a month or more in doses exceeding two to three times the single hypnotic dose (400 to 600 mg. per day), a major withdrawal syndrome will not develop.

Table 6.1 summarizes the results of experimental studies on physical dependence in humans produced by several common sedative-hypnotics. All the studies involved major symptoms of withdrawal such as seizures or psychosis.

DETOXIFICATION

Although the physically dependent individual must go through detoxification or withdrawal at some point during any drug abuse treatment regimen, it is not necessarily the first step. Drug abusers frequently request detoxification

Table 6.1 Dosages of Selected Sedative-hypnotics Producing Physical Dependence

Drug	Dosage needed to produce dependence (mg./day)	Time required for dependence to develop (in days)	Time required for convulsions to occur after withdrawal is initiated (in days)
Secobarbital and pentobarbital	800–2,200	35–37	2–3
Diazepam	80–120	42	5–8
Chlordiazepoxide	300–600	60–180	5–8
Meprobamate	2,400	—	2–3

Source: Essig, 1964; Hollister, Motzenbecker, and Degan, 1961; Hollister et al., 1963; Wikler, 1955.

services because they believe that the treatment facility expects it of them rather than because they actually want to be withdrawn from a particular drug. Many request treatment during a psychological, social, or personal crisis. Although this is an ideal time to utilize crisis intervention techniques, it is not necessarily the most auspicious time to begin withdrawal, which generates additional psychological and physiological stress in the individual. It is often better to "stabilize" the individual's pattern of drug use first and then attempt to resolve the crises that led him to therapy rather than to initiate withdrawal immediately.

The goal of drug detoxification is the safe, comfortable treatment of physical dependence. If a patient is comfortably and completely withdrawn from a drug, the withdrawal phase of treatment should be regarded as successful, even if the individual resumes his drug use immediately after treatment. There are two major methods of detoxifying the patient who is physically dependent on barbiturates: (1) gradual withdrawal of the addicting agent and (2) the substitution of phenobarbital for the addicting agent and gradual withdrawal of the substitute drug.

Withdrawal of Addicting Agent

Traditionally, withdrawal from barbiturates is accomplished with the barbiturate of addiction in amounts that produce mild toxicity (Isbell, 1950). Step-by-step withdrawal of the barbiturate should generally proceed at a rate no greater than 100 mg. per day. Data derived from sleep research indicates that even at this rate, rebound of REM sleep occurs. This phenomenon is reported clinically as nightmares and increasingly vivid dreams. To avoid sleep disturbances, the rate of withdrawal should probably be slower (Kales et al., 1970; Wikler, 1968).

In our early clinical experience with barbiturate withdrawal, we found that withdrawal with short-acting barbiturates was difficult to control. The dosage differential between mild toxicity and disinhibition was only one to two pills per day, and our patients often became behavioral problems on the ward. It was this complication that led us to seek a different method of withdrawal.

Substitution Technique

Although phenobarbital was employed sporadically as a treatment agent for barbiturate and other sedative-hypnotic withdrawal as early as 1951 (Alexander, 1951; Goldman & Ulett, 1968; Wulff, 1959), the *techniques* for using the drug were not standardized or systematically tested in a clinical setting on a large number of patients until the late 1960s (e.g., Smith, Wesson & Lannon, 1969; Smith & Wesson, 1970).

The rationale for the phenobarbital substitution technique is similar to the rationale for substituting methadone for heroin. The longer acting agent permits a withdrawal characterized by fewer fluctuations in blood levels of the drug throughout the day and thus enables the safe use of smaller doses. The safety factor for phenobarbital is greater than that for the shorter acting barbiturates; lethal doses of phenobarbital are several times greater than toxic doses and the signs of toxicity (e.g., sustained nystagmus, slurred speech, and ataxia) are easy to observe. And finally, because phenobarbital intoxication usually does not produce disinhibition, the behavioral problems commonly associated with the short-acting barbiturates seldom occur.

During the first two days, the individual is transferred to a stabilizing dose of phenobarbital. Ordinarily, no drugs other than phenobarbital are used. In an experimental study of barbiturate withdrawal in dogs, Essig and Carter (1962) found that diphenylhydantoin (Dilantin®) was not an effective anticonvulsant, even when administered intravenously. Essig and Fraser (1966) later discovered that dogs treated with a placebo had the same number of withdrawal seizures as those treated with chlorpromazine (Thorazine®).

The dosage of phenobarbital is calculated by substituting one *sedative dose* (30 mg.) of phenobarbital for each *hypnotic dose* (100 mg.) of the short-acting barbiturate the patient has been using, up to 600 mg. of phenobarbital per day. Despite the fact that many addicts exaggerate the magnitude of their addiction, we find that a patient's history is the best guide when initiating withdrawal. If he has grossly overstated the extent of his addiction, toxic symptoms will appear within a day or two after treatment is initiated. This problem is easily managed by omitting one or more doses of phenobarbital and recalculating the daily dosage.

If the patient shows signs of withdrawal—such as anxiety, sleep disturbance, orthostatic hypotension, hyperreflexia, muscle twitches, or stomach cramps—he is given 200 mg. of phenobarbital intramuscularly, and his total daily dose of phenobarbital is increased by 25 per cent. Should he show signs of phenobarbital toxicity (sustained nystagmus, slurred speech, or staggering gait), his daily dosage is reduced by half and withdrawal proceeds.

Some clinicians use a pentobarbital challenge to establish the degree of tolerance and physical dependence on a barbiturate. This technique involves the intramuscular injection of 200 mg. of pentobarbital; the patient is then observed for signs of toxicity. The absence of nystagmus, unsteady gait, and slurred speech is accepted as evidence of significant tolerance and presumed physical dependency. Signs of toxicity are accepted as presumptive evidence against tolerance and physical dependency. We have found that the phenobarbital substitution technique makes this diagnostic test unnecessary in most cases.

The phenobarbital substitution technique can also be used with short-acting sedative-hypnotics other than barbiturates. Table 6.2 lists the equivalent of phenobarbital used to withdraw patients from the barbiturates and a variety of other sedative-hypnotics.

Table 6.2   Phenobarbital Withdrawal Equivalents for Common Sedative-hypnotics

Drug	Dosage (in mg.)	Phenobarbital Withdrawal Equivalent (mg.)
Barbiturates		
Amobarbital	100	30
Butabarbital	60	30
Pentobarbital	100	30
Secobarbital	100	30
Other sedative-hypnotics		
Chloral hydrate	500	30
Ethchlorvynol (Placidyl®)	350	30
Glutethimide (Doriden®)	250	30
Meprobamate (Equanil®, Miltown®)	400	30
Methaqualone (Quaalude®, Sopor®, etc.)	300	30
Methyprylon (Noludar®)	100	30
Benzodiazepines		
Chlordiazepoxide (Librium®)	100	30
Clorazepate (Tranxene®)	50	30
Diazepam (Valium®)	50	30
Flurazepam (Dalmane®)	30	30
Oxazepam (Serax®)	100	30

Source: Wesson and Smith, 1974, p. 165.

PHYSICAL DEPENDENCY IN INFANTS

Because barbiturates cross the placental barrier, there is always the chance that the signs of physical dependence will occur in the neonate of a mother who is physically dependent upon barbiturates. Cases of neonatal physical dependence on barbiturates began to appear in the literature in the early 1970s (Bleyer & Marshall, 1972; Desmond et al., 1972). The onset of withdrawal symptoms may not occur until the infant has left the hospital; the median onset of symptoms is seven days. The functional immaturity of the neonate's liver and kidneys may be a factor in the slow onset of withdrawal symptoms. (The signs and symptoms of heroin and barbiturate withdrawal in neonates and adults are contrasted in Table 6.3.)

Table 6.3 Signs and Symptoms of Withdrawal from Heroin and Barbiturates in Adults and Infants

Drug	Signs and symptoms of withdrawal	
	In adults	*In infants*
Heroin	Anxiety	Irritability
	Runny nose	Hyperactivity
	Dilated pupils	Tremulousness
	Cramps	Poor food intake
	Diarrhea, vomiting	Diarrhea, vomiting
	Shaking chills	Fever
	Profuse sweating	High-pitched cry
	Sleep disturbances	Disturbed sleep
	Aches and pains	Hyperreflexia
		Major motor seizures
Barbiturates	Anxiety	High-pitched cry
	Irritability	Tremors
	Restlessness	Restlessness
	Sleep disturbances	Disturbed sleep
	Postural hypotension	Hyperreflexia
	Delirium	Hyperphagia
	Hyperpyrexia	Diarrhea, vomiting
	Major motor seizures	Major motor seizures

When an infant is diagnosed as suffering from barbiturate withdrawal, treatment with phenobarbital should begin immediately. Because of the gastrointestinal upset related to withdrawal, the first doses should be administered intramuscularly. An initial dose of 10 to 12 mg. per kilogram of body weight should be given; the amount should then be tapered off over a period of at least one month (Bleyer & Marshall, 1972; Freeman, 1970, Desmond et al., 1972).

Although physical dependence on barbiturates should be considered in instances of neonatal seizures, seizures can also be related to a variety of other conditions. Freeman (1970), for example, cites the following possible causes:

Aminoaciduria: phenylketonuria, maple sugar urine disease, hyperglycemia

Anoxia

Birth trauma

Developmental anomalies: cerebral dysgenesis, incontinentia pigmenti

Drug withdrawal: heroin, alcohol, barbiturates

Encephalitis

Hypocalcemia

Hypoglycemia

Hypomagnesemia

Hyponatremia or hypernatremia

Kernicterus

Meningitis

Pyridoxine (B6) disorders

Sepsis

DEPENDENCE ON MIXED DRUGS

Alcohol and Sedative-hypnotics

The individual who uses only one sedative-hypnotic, e.g, secobarbital, is relatively rare. Most abusers use a variety of sedative-hypnotics, either separately or in combination with alcohol. In our research on polydrug abuse, we have tried to eliminate patients whose primary drug of addiction is alcohol; yet we find that 15 per cent of the individuals who request treatment for barbiturate dependency also exhibit diagnostic criteria for alcoholism.

Management of a dual dependence on alcohol and sedative-hypnotics is similar to the management of dependencies on other sedative-hypnotics. Because sedative-hypnotics and alcohol are cross tolerant, phenobarbital will substitute for alcohol as well as for sedative-hypnotics. Thus when determining the appropriate dosages for withdrawal, it is important to know whether the patient has been using alcohol concurrently with the sedative-hypnotics or has been using the two separately. Some individuals prefer barbiturates but will switch to alcohol when barbiturates are unavailable. Others use both drugs simultaneously. If the two are used together, the physician must consider their additive effect on the degree of physical dependency when calculating the initial dose of phenobarbital. We substitute 15 mg. of phenobarbital for each 30 cc. of 80- to 100-proof alcohol. We then add it to the amount of phenobarbital we have determined is necessary to treat withdrawal from the sedative-hypnotic. The following case history illustrates this technique:

> A 53-year-old man contacted us because of his combined alcohol/barbiturate dependency. He suffered from chronic insomnia and had begun taking secobarbital and pentobarbital to induce sleep. He had also used alcohol excessively several times during his life and had been diagnosed as an alcoholic. On admission, he told us that to sleep, he had to take 300 to 600 mg. of barbiturates and one-half to two-thirds of a fifth of 80-proof vodka. We calculated the medication for withdrawal on the basis of the following alcohol/phenobarbital equivalents:

1 ounce	80-proof alcohol =	30 cc. =	15 mg. phenobarbital
1 pint	80-proof alcohol =	480 cc. =	240 mg. phenobarbital
1 fifth (4/5 qt)	80-proof alcohol =	760 cc. =	380 mg. phenobarbital
1 quart	80-proof alcohol =	960 cc. =	480 mg. phenobarbital

> Thus one-half a fifth of 80-proof vodka is equivalent to 190 mg. of phenobarbital, or ½ X 380 mg. = 190 mg. Because 600 mg. of secobarbital is equivalent to 180 mg. of phenobarbital and the effects of sedative-hypnotics are additive, the alcohol equivalent (190 mg.) and secobarbital equivalent (180 mg.) of phenobarbital would total 370 mg.

Opiates and Sedative-hypnotics

Sedative-hypnotics and heroin can be abused concurrently in amounts large enough to produce physical dependence on both. Furthermore, individuals on methadone maintenance can also develop a dependence on sedative-hypnotics.

Because the symptoms of withdrawal from opiates and barbiturates are similar, the clinical picture is difficult to assess when both drugs are withdrawn at the same time. In general, it is preferable to withdraw the sedative-hypnotic first, preventing opiate withdrawal by using methadone to maintain the patient. When the patient is barbiturate free, the methadone can be withdrawn at a rate of 5 mg. per day.

Chapter 7

NONMEDICAL ASPECTS OF
BARBITURATE ABUSE

So far, we have focused primarily on the acute medical treatment and detoxification of the barbiturate abuser. In this final chapter, we will briefly discuss issues related to long-term treatment of barbiturate abusers, control of barbiturate availability, and the impact of barbiturates on society.

AFTERCARE

In most cases, medical treatment alone will not sufficiently alter an individual life-style that revolves around the excessive use of sedative-hypnotics. Thus after a barbiturate abuser has been detoxified and his medical disorders have been treated, the physician should reevaluate the patient carefully to determine his additional needs. This evaluative process can begin early in the detoxification phase of treatment so that the patient's transition into long-term treatment will proceed as smoothly as possible.

Because of the wide variety of patterns and motivations for barbiturate use, no single treatment plan will be applicable to all barbiturate abusers. Adequate treatment is based on careful evaluation of individual patients, and interventions are selected on the basis of individual needs.

The vast majority of research on aftercare of drug abusers has been conducted in the area of heroin abuse; only recently have efforts been made to design aftercare programs specifically for those who abuse nonnarcotic or mixed drugs (Smith, Wesson & Lerner, 1974). The technology for aftercare of the nonnarcotic barbiturate user is still primitive. No systematic research has focused on how barbiturate abusers respond to different treatment interventions. As a result, most clinicians in the field rely on their personal experience when treating barbiturate abusers.

The two major methods of treating heroin addicts following crisis intervention and detoxification are methadone maintenance and therapeutic communities (Senay & Renault, 1971). Because methadone is a long-acting oral narcotic that effectively blocks only the effects of narcotics, it is not useful in the treatment of barbiturate dependence. However, with appropriate diagnoses, other forms of psychopharmacological treatment can be useful. For example, when an individual abuses barbiturates to self-medicate episodes of hyperactivity, lithium can be useful to stabilize his mood. After detoxification, a careful evaluation may determine that a patient is suffering a major thought disorder which might respond to treatment with the phenothiazine tranquilizers.

The rate of recidivism among detoxified barbiturate abusers who were self-medicating an underlying depression has been reduced by careful use of tricyclic antidepressants in conjunction with individual or group counseling and psychotherapy. Nonpharmacological treatment modalities such as Transcendental Meditation (Marcus, 1975) and biofeedback training appear to be promising treatment techniques for selected patients.

In our experience, the therapeutic community that developed in the area of heroin abuse has proved to be largely inappropriate for the barbiturate or nonnarcotic polydrug abuser (Smith et al., 1974). Many traditional treatment modalities that were designed to care for the heroin addict are relatively limited in terms of their applicability to other drug problems, especially those that involve severe psychopathology. However, there are some promising lines of inquiry.

Some patients who abuse barbiturates are receptive to individual psychotherapy after detoxification. The emphasis on family therapy is also increasing (Hirsch & Imhof, 1975), and some barbiturate abusers we have detoxified have benefited from the nonstressful, structured, supportive, work-oriented environment provided in day care programs sponsored by community mental health centers.

One difficulty in attempting to design a long-term treatment plan for the heavy user of sedative-hypnotics is the cerebral dysfunction that persists after detoxification (Adams et al., 1975; Judd & Grant, 1975). For example, some users have difficulty in abstract thinking and in performing tasks that require complex perceptual and motor skills. These individuals do not benefit from insight-oriented psychotherapy and may be too fragile for encounter groups. Thus rehabilitation efforts with these patients may have to be directed toward maximizing their intact adaptive abilities while reducing expectations concerning abilities that are impaired. After several months of abstinence from drugs, some of their cerebral dysfunction will clear up, and the treatment plan can then be modified: e.g., psychotherapy can become more insight-oriented and higher level vocational rehabilitation efforts can be instituted. During long-term treatment of the sedative-hypnotic abuser, his psychological status should be reassessed periodically and the treatment plan should be modified accordingly.

ATTITUDES OF THE MEDICAL PROFESSION

Many physicians have an extremely negative attitude about drug abusers, and this attitude is reflected in hospital policies. We frequently have to admit barbiturate abusers to hospitals for detoxification under the guise of seizure disorder or some other confounding diagnoses because of hospital policies against the treatment of drug addicts under any circumstances. The necessity for hiding the primary diagnosis, of course, goes far beyond barbiturate abuse; it also crops up with other forms of drug abuse including alcoholism.

AVAILABILITY OF BARBITURATES

Congressional hearings on barbiturates held in 1971 and 1972 focused primarily on the quantities of legitimately manufactured barbiturates that reach the black market and the persons who are responsible for this diversion (Subcommittee to Investigate Juvenile Delinquency, 1972). Diversion can occur at any point in the chain of warehousing, distribution, and dispensing of legitimate drugs. The more common methods are hijacking and theft; spurious orders from nonexistent firms; illicit sales by wholesalers, retailers, or physicians; small-scale pilfering from family medicine chests; and the sale of drugs obtained with legitimate or forged prescriptions.

Illicit Sources

At present, there is no evidence that any barbiturates are manufactured illegally in the United States. However, in 1974 the Comptroller General of the United States indicated that the amount of barbiturates produced illegally in Mexico is increasing. In 1972 the Mexican government seized three laboratories that reportedly produced and exported six million doses of barbiturates and amphetamines to the United States. In late 1974 it was estimated that about three million tablets of dangerous drugs (including both barbiturates and amphetamines) come from Mexico each year.

Figure 7.1 illustrates in graphic form our analysis of the illegal sources, distribution, and production of barbiturates in the United States. Each X enclosed in a circle indicates possible points where diversion takes place. In essence, any time bulk quantities of drugs are shipped from one point to another, there is the possibility that part or all of the shipment will be diverted to the black market.

Small-scale diversions such as forged prescriptions and burglaries of drugstores, warehouses, and physicians' offices, account for a substantial portion of black market barbiturates, as do "patients" who go from physician to physician obtaining prescriptions for barbiturates.

The capsule containing barbiturates obtained in the black market—even if it carries an identifiable brand name —may not accurately reflect its contents. These capsules are often refilled either with diluted barbiturates or another substance. For example, one study of black market secobarbital "reds" found that the contents varied between 21 to more than 100 mg. per capsule (Finkle, 1971).

Because barbiturates diverted from legitimate sources are frequently repackaged in nondescript capsules, drug companies and law enforcement agencies draw the erroneous conclusion that these barbiturates were manufactured

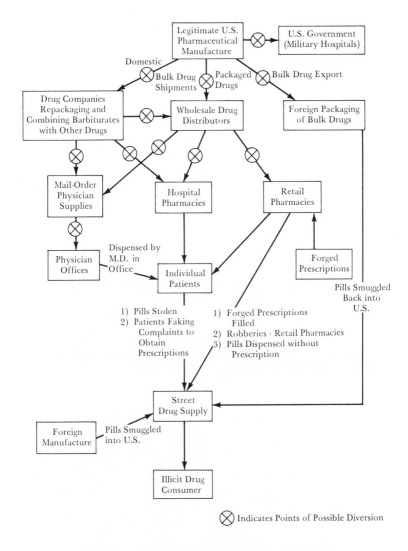

Figure 7.1 Routes by which barbiturates reach the black market (Smith & Wesson, 1973, p. 110).

and packaged illicitly. A complex case involving a pharmacist at a large hospital in southern California illustrates how this confusion can arise.

> A 32-year-old pharmacist had a grand mal seizure in the hospital parking lot and was taken to the emergency room, where he was treated with short-acting barbitures. Based on his answers to interrogation by police and representatives of the American Pharmaceutical Association, it was determined that he ingested approximately 30 to 40 capsules (each containing 100 mg.) of Seconal® (secobarbital) per day and experienced the seizure while attempting to reduce his habit because of the difficulties he was having in obtaining his usual supply.
>
> The pharmacist ordered secobarbital in large quantities from wholesale drug catalogs using the hospital's stationery. When Seconal® was delivered to the hospital pharmacy, he would steal several hundred capsules at a time. He would then purchase standard, unmarked red gelatin capsules and repackage the stolen Seconal®, put approximately 50 mg. in each capsule and keep the remaining 50 mg. for himself. He would then sell the unmarked capsules on the street as street "reds" containing 100 mg. of secobarbital. Because these capsules were unmarked, both law enforcement officials and the manufacturer erroneously assumed that the drug was not of domestic origin. In addition to selling barbiturates directly to street dealers, the pharmacist used them to obtain sexual services from young girls who were barbiturate users.
>
> As a result of these complex machinations, the pharmacist was able to generate substantial extra income as well as supply his escalating barbiturate habit. As his thefts became larger, however, the hospital administration began to suspect that the thefts were occurring on the premises. When the pharmacist attempted to reduce the size of his habit to avoid detection, he had the seizure. However, he had avoided detection for two years, and it is unlikely that the police ever would have discovered his illegal activities had his seizure not focused attention on him.

Role of Physicians and the Pharmaceutical Industry

Much of the testimony presented at the congressional hearings on barbiturates by the Pharmaceutical Manufacturers'

Association and the American Medical Association in the early 1970s was designed to extricate the physician and the pharmaceutical industry from responsibility for barbiturate abuse (Subcommittee to Investigate Juvenile Delinquency, 1972). This was unfortunate because the precise roles that the pharmaceutical industry and physicians *do* play in contributing to the black market supply of barbiturates should be delineated.

Figure 7.1 indicates that physicians are responsible for the diversion far down the diversion chain. Some of this diversion is related to poor prescribing practices or to misguided attempts to provide legitimate care. A few physicians deliberately contribute to the black market for their own personal gain. The distribution of illicitly manufactured drugs via the black market and the distribution of legally manufactured drugs through medical channels must be analyzed as separate phenomena in considering control strategies.

Control Measures

The quantities of barbiturates that find their way through each channel to the black market are impossible to determine at present. Any attempt to control the flow through one channel must take into consideration the possible consequences on other routes of diversion and procurement. If, for example, the supply diverted from legitimate domestic sources is effectively controlled, increasing quantities may reach the black market from foreign sources or from illicit domestic sources. In other words, controls alone will not eliminate abuse of barbiturates since the same rules of supply and demand apply to the barbiturates as to any other commodity. A decreased supply in the face of continued demand will result in an increase in price. When the price becomes high enough, industrious entrepreneurs will enter the field and generate new sources of supply.

In November 1973 amobarbital, secobarbital, and

pentobarbital (excluding suppository forms) were moved to Schedule II of the Controlled Substances Act. Other barbiturates are currently controlled under Schedules III or IV. Production quotas can be established for Schedule II drugs, as was done for amphetamines in 1972. However, critics of production control doubt that decreasing the supply of legitimate drugs will decrease the amount of abuse significantly. As evidence, they point to the continued abuse of heroin despite the fact that the drug is not produced legally. Furthermore, quotas will mean that legitimate consumers will have to pay more for barbiturates because of increased amount of paperwork that will be required of drug manufacturers, wholesalers, pharmacists, and physicians.

SOCIAL AND ECONOMIC CONSIDERATIONS

The social cost of barbiturate abuse is similar to the cost of alcohol abuse rather than heroin abuse. Medical complications, accidents, and overdoses require expensive medical management and hospitalization. Loss of productivity, disrupted families, and judgmental errors also have their social cost, although measuring these social factors in economic terms is more complex. Although many heroin addicts are motivated to seek treatment because they object to the constant activity required to support their expensive habits, barbiturate abusers rarely experience these economic pressures.

Barbiturate intoxication is relatively inexpensive to achieve, compared with heroin. An intoxicating dose of heroin costs eight to ten times as much as an intoxicating dose of barbiturates. The cost of intoxicating doses of alcohol and barbiturates is similar if the barbiturates are purchased singly in the black market. Because drug users usually purchase in quantity, thereby reducing the cost per unit, barbiturate intoxication is within reach of most teen-agers and young adults. The cost factor is probably one reason why barbiturates are so popular among clients in methadone maintenance programs who supplement their methadone with barbiturates or other sedative-hypnotics.

Cost is not the only reason that teen-agers prefer barbiturates. Unlike alcohol, barbiturates are easy to carry, can be swallowed unobtrusively, and leave no distinctive odor on the breath or clothing. Some teen-agers have a free source of barbiturates because their parents are unlikely to notice that half-a-dozen capsules have disappeared from a bottle containing 50 or 100 capsules.

Because the barbiturate addict, unlike the heroin addict, is seldom forced to steal or commit other crimes to pay for his drugs, the social cost of barbiturate abuse is less obvious than that of heroin abuse and has received far less attention. We believe, however, that the cost of barbiturate abuse is substantial when all its ramifications are considered. This cost is measured in terms of overdoses, medical complications, family disruption, and unnecessary use of emergency rooms and psychiatric services. The treatment of physical dependency also expends medical resources that could perhaps be better spent elsewhere.

On the other hand, the benefits of access to sedative-hypnotics are more difficult to measure. Using barbiturates to alleviate the emotional stress related to psychological trauma, or to obtain a good night's sleep during severe stress no doubt enhances the capacity of many individuals to function in a variety of settings. We do not necessarily accept the premise that the opportunity for psychothera-peutic resolution is necessarily squelched by alleviating psychic distress with sedatives. In many cases, the situation is temporary, the stresses are rooted in reality, and the individual may not be in a position to benefit from insight-oriented psychotherapy. Only to the extent that phar-maceutical solutions rob the individual who is otherwise motivated for psychotherapy and is capable of psychotherapeutic resolution of problems are chemical solutions malevolent.

SUMMARY

With this book, we have tried to supply a rational perspective on the use and abuse of barbiturates. We devoted more pages to barbiturate abuse and its associated consequences than to legitimate medical usage, in part, because we did not include a detailed discussion about important uses of barbiturates in anesthesia but instead referred the reader to an excellent book by Dundee and Wyant (1974).

Fortunately, the barbiturates that are currently abused most often are the ones which are most medically expendable. Three barbiturates—secobarbital, pentobarbital, and amobarbital—account for most cases of abuse. Their clinical use is indicated primarily for the treatment of insomnia. In most instances, the benzodiazepine hypnotics are at least of equal effectiveness, they appear to have less potential for abuse, and they are safer if ingested in excessive quantities. The fact that the number of prescriptions written for the barbiturates is declining reflects in large part a shift toward the benzodiazepines. Currently, the advantages of barbiturates over the benzodiazepines are (1) the lower unit-dosage-cost of barbiturates, (2) most physicians are familiar with barbiturates, and (3) barbiturates are listed on the formularies of publicly funded medical assistance programs. The major disadvantages of barbiturates are (1) REM suppression with a resulting rebound when the drug is stopped—a contributing factor to the development of physiological dependence, (2) their popularity as recreational drugs, (3) their solubility, which encourages a pattern of intravenous use, (4) their capacity to induce liver enzyme production, which results in increased metabolism of other drugs, and (5) their lethality when taken in over-dose quantities. The incidence of adverse reactions to both the barbiturates and benzodiazepines is low when either drug is taken in normally prescribed dosages.

With the exception of the benzodiazepines, "minor tranquilizers" promoted as lacking the disadvantages of barbiturates do not offer any special therapeutic advantages. In our opinion, some minor tranquilizers such as gluthethimide (Doriden®) are even more toxic than the barbiturates when taken in overdose quantities.

Pentobarbital, secobarbital, and amobarbital are not indispensable to the practice of medicine just because millions of doses are prescribed each year. Most physicians would not have a strong preference for prescribing barbiturates over the benzodiazepines if the latter cost less and were listed on the formularies of hospitals and public medical care programs.

Although barbiturate abuse is a problem of considerable magnitude, much of that problem would not cease to exist if barbiturates were suddenly removed from the American market. If the demand for barbiturates was great enough, illicit domestic manufacturing would be stimulated and complicate the problem of control still further. Most barbiturates abused in the context of the street drug scene are brought into the country illicitly. The abuse of prescription-originated barbiturates would probably be affected to a greater extent if barbiturates were withdrawn from the legitimate market. Many patients would probably turn to other sedative-hypnotics including the benzodiazepines and alcohol.

Knowledge about the treatment of individuals who have developed a pattern of chronic intoxication with barbiturates is still in its infancy. Basic research into the biochemistry of barbiturate dependence is needed. As outlined in Chapter 6, the treatment of physical dependence on barbiturates is well developed at the clinical level and is usually successful when the patient will cooperate. Postdetoxification treatment, however, is still unsuccessful in many cases.

Although some patients who use barbiturates to cover or self-medicate severe depression or schizophrenia can be treated definitively with antidepressants or phenothiazines, our experience indicates that relatively few individuals prefer these agents to their barbiturate of choice. Those who undertake the treatment of a chronic barbiturate abuser must be prepared for episodic relapses and be flexible in their treatment strategies. In our work with individuals who have developed a pattern of chronic intoxication, we have been impressed by the difficulties of attempting insight-oriented psychotherapeutic interventions and the necessity for modifying the abuser's social environment as part of the therapeutic strategy.

Treatment modalities such as biofeedback and acupuncture may offer some promise for treating selected individuals, but they have not been tested in systematically controlled studies with barbiturate abusers. And pharmacological treatment with sedatives of any class is generally contraindicated because individuals who are dependent on one sedative are likely to escalate the dosage of any sedative prescribed. Teaching drug abusers how to cope with everyday anxieties without resorting to pharmacological oblivion is a long, arduous process.

APPENDIXES

A

Generic, Chemical, and Trade Names of the Barbiturates

The literature yields a bewildering variety of barbiturate names, partly because of the different trade names and partly because the terminology varies from country to country. The following list catalogs the more commonly encountered names for the barbiturates.

Generic name	Chemical name	Other trade and generic names
allobarbital	5,5-diallylbarbituric acid	allbarbital allobarbitone Diadol
amobarbital	5-ethyl-5-isopentyl barbituric acid, or 5-ethyl-5-isoamyl-barbituric acid	amylobarbitone (U.K.) Amytal (U.K.) allional
aprobarbital	5-allyl-5-isopropylbarbituric acid	Allonal allylisopropylbar- bituric acid Allylpropymal allypropymal Alurate Aprozal Isonal (Swedish) Numal Somnipron Verdum
barbital	5,5-diethylbarbituric acid or sodium 5,5-diethyl-barbiturate	barbitone (U.K.) diemal diethylbarbiturate monosodium diethylbarbituric acid diethylmalonylurea Veronal

Generic name	Chemical name	Other trade and generic names
butalbital	5-allyl-5-isobutylbarbituric acid	allylbarbitone allylbarbituric acid allylisobutyl barbiturate allylisobutyl-barbituric acid Sandoptal
butallylonal	5-(2-bromoallyl)-5-*sec*-butyl-barbituric acid	butallylonal Pernocton Pernoston
cyclobarbital	5-(1-cyclohexen-1-yl)-5-ethylbarbituric acid	cyclobarbitone Phanodorm Phanodorn
mephobarbital	5-ethyl-1-methyl-5-phenyl-barbituric acid	Mebaral Menta-Bal Mephoral phemitone (U.K.) Prominal (U.K.)
methohexital	5-allyl-(1-methyl-2-pentynylbarbituric acid	Brietal Brevital methohexitone (U.K.)
pentobarbital	5-ethyl-5-(1-methylbutyl) barbituric acid	Aquabarb Nembutal pentobarbitone (U.K.) Pentosol
phenobarbital	5-ethyl-5-phenylbarbituric acid	Eskabarb Lixophen Luminal phenobarbitone (U.K.) Phenoturic phenylethylbarbituric acid phenylethylmalony-lurea Solu-Barb Stental
probarbital	5-ethyl-5-isopropyl-barbituric acid	Ipral probarbital
secobarbital	5-allyl-5-(1-methylbutyl) barbituric acid	quinalbarbitone secobarbitone (U.K.) Seconal
thiamylal	5-allyl-5-(1-methylbutyl)-2-thiobarbituric acid	Surital Hipnopento
thiopental	5-ethyl-5-(1-methylbutyl)-2-thiobarbituric acid	Intraval Pentothal thiopentone (U.K.)

B

Street Terms for Barbiturates and Other Drugs

There are numerous street names for barbiturates. Secobarbital, for example, which is generally packaged in red or
pink capsules, is called any of the following names: F-40s,
Mexican reds, M & Ms, R.D.s, red birds, red bullets, red
devils, red dolls, red lillies, reds, seccies, or seggies. Pentobarbital, usually a yellow capsule, is called nebbies, nem-
bies, yellow bullets, yellow dolls, yellow jackets, or yellows.
Capsules containing equal parts of secobarbital and amobarbital are common and are known as double trouble,
gorilla pills, rainbows, reds and blues, tootsies, trees, or
tuies. Drugs that are available on the street are not necessarily of pharmaceutical quality. Any red or pink pill containing a barbiturate may be called Seconal®, much the
same way as any cola drink is called Coca-Cola, and products in a capsule bearing a pharmaceutical company's
trademark may have been repackaged. The following contains the street names of a number of drugs:

Street terms	Drug
Abbotts	Nembutal (sodium pentobarbital) capsules
Backwards	Tranquilizers or barbiturates; to get a habit again; to backslide
Barb freak	Intravenous barbiturate user
Barbs	Barbiturates
Blockbusters	Barbiturates; Nembutal (sodium pentobarbital) capsules
Blue angels, bluebirds, blue bullets, blue devils, blue dolls, blue heavens, blues, blue tips	Amobarbital or Amytal capsules
Candy	Barbiturates; any drug you like
Christmas trees	Dexamyl capsules (dextroamphetamine sulfate and amobarbital).

121

Street terms	Drug
Dolls	Barbiturates
Double trouble	Capsules containing sodium secobarbital and sodium amobarbital; Tuinal; also generic products
Down	Barbiturates or any sedative drug; also a depressed state, sometimes related to intoxication but also to the absence of drugs
F-40s	Seconal (sodium secobarbital) capsules
G.B.s	Barbiturates; goofballs
Geronimo	Alcohol mixed with barbiturates
Goofballs	Barbiturates
Goofers	Barbiturates; Doriden (glutethimide)
Gorilla pills	Capsules containing sodium secobarbital and sodium amobarbital); Tuinal; available as generic products
Hearts	Amphetamines; Dexamyl (dextroamphetamine sulfate and amobarbital) tablets
Idiot pills	Barbiturates
King Kong pills	Barbiturates
Mexican reds	Any red capsule containing sodium secobarbital (Seconal)
Mother's little helper	Meprobamate (Miltown, Equanil)
Nebbies, nembies, nemmies	Nembutal (sodium pentobarbital) capsules
Peanuts	Barbiturates
Phennies	Phenobarbital tablets
Pillhead	Habitual user of barbiturates or amphetamines
Pink ladies	Barbiturates
Pinks	Any pinkish capsule containing sodium secobarbital (Seconal)
Purple hearts	Dexamyl (dextroamphetamine sulfate and amobarbital) tablets
Rainbows	See gorilla pills
R.D.s, reds, red birds, red bullets, red devils, red dolls	Any red capsule containing secobarbital (Seconal)
Reds and blues	See gorilla pills
Seccies, seggies	Seconal (sodium secobarbital) capsules
Sleepers, softballs, stumblers	Downers, barbiturates, any central nervous system depressant
Tootsies, trees, tuies	Tuinal (sodium secobarbital and sodium amobarbital) capsules
Wallbanger	Someone showing lack of muscular coordination caused by intoxication with sedative-hypnotics or alcohol
Yellow bullets, yellow dolls, yellow jackets, yellows	Any yellow capsule containing pentobarbital (Nembutal)

REFERENCES

Adams, K. M., Rennick, P. M., Schooff, K. G., & Keegan, J. F. Neuropsychological measurement of drug effects: Polydrug research. *Journal for Psychedelic Drugs*, 1975, **7**(2), 151–160.

Alexander, E. J. Withdrawal effects of sodium amytal. *Diseases of the Nervous System*, 1951, **12**, 77–82.

American Medical Association. *Drug evaluations* (2nd ed.) Acton, Mass.: Publishing Sciences Group, 1973.

American Medical Association. Failure to diagnose barbiturate intoxication. *The Citation*, 1971, **24**, 22–23.

Aserinsky, E., & Kleitman, N. Regularly occurring periods of eye motility, and concomitant phenomena, during sleep. *Science*, 1953, **118**, 273–274.

Baeyer, A. Untersuchungen über die Harnsäuregruppe. *Justus Liebig's Annalen der Chemie und Pharmacie*, 1863, **127**, 230–236.

Birch, C. A. Jaundice due to phenobarbital. *Lancet*, 1936, **1**, 478–479.

Bleckwenn, W. J. Production of sleep and rest in psychotic cases: A preliminary report. *Archives of Neurology and Psychiatry*, 1930, **24**, 365–372.

Bleyer, W. A., & Marshall, R. E. Barbiturate withdrawal syndrome in a passively addicted infant. *Journal of the American Medical Association*, 1972, **221**, 185–186.

Breckenridge, A., & Orme, M. Interaction of benzodiazepines with oral anticoagulants. In S. Garattini, E. Mussini, & Randall, L. O. (Eds.), *The benzodiazepines.* New York: Raven Press, 1973.

Brown, S. S., Lyons, S. M., & Dundee, J. W. Intra-arterial barbiturates: A study of some factors leading to intravascular thrombosis. *British Journal of Anaesthesia*, 1968, **40**, 13–19.

Catlin, D. H. *A guide to urine testing for drugs of abuse. Special Action Office Monograph*, Series B, No. 2, 1973.

Chambers, C. D. Barbiturate-sedative abuse: A study of prevalence among narcotic abusers. *International Journal of the Addictions*, 1969, **4**, 45–57.

Cohen, S. M. Accidental intra-arterial injection of drugs. *Lancet*, 1948, **255**, 361–371.

Committee on Alcoholism and Addiction and Council on Mental Health. Dependence on barbiturates and other sedative drugs. *Journal of the American Medical Association*, 1965, **193**, 673–677.

Committee on Alcoholism and Drug Dependence. Barbiturate and barbiturate like drugs. *Journal of the American Medical Association*, 1974, **230**, 1440–1441.

Comptroller General of the United States. *Efforts to stop narcotics and dangerous drugs coming from and through Mexico and Central America.* (GAO Publication No. GGD-75-44), Washington, D.C.: December 31, 1974.

Cumberlidge, M. C. The abuse of barbiturates by heroin addicts. *Canadian Medical Association Journal*, 1968, **98**, 1045–1049.

Curran, F. J. The symptoms and treatment of barbiturate intoxication and psychosis. *American Journal of Psychiatry*, 1938, **95**, 73–81.

Dean, G. Porphyria. *British Medical Journal*, 1953, **2**, 1291–1294.

Dement, W. The effect of dream deprivation. *Science*, 1960, **131**, 1705–1707.

Dement, W., & Kleitman, N. Cyclic variations in EEG during sleep and their relation to eye movements, body motility, and dreaming. *Electroencephalography and Clinical Neurophysiology*, 1957, **9**, 673–690.

Desmond, M. M., Schwanecke, R. P., Wilson, G. S., Yasunaga, S., & Burgdorff, I. Maternal barbiturate utilization and neonatal withdrawal symptomatology. *Journal of Pediatrics*, 1972, **80**, 190–197.

Domestic Council Drug Abuse Task Force. *White paper on drug abuse: September, 1975.* Washington, D.C.: U.S. Government Printing Office, 1975.

Dorpat, T. L. Drug automatism, barbiturate poisoning, and suicide behavior. *Archives of General Psychiatry*, 1974, **31**, 216–220.

Dox, A. W., & Yoder, L. Some derivatives of normal-butyl-malonic acid. *Journal of the American Chemical Society*, 1922, **44**, 1578–1581.

Drugs for epilepsy. *The Medical Letter*, 1976, **18**(6), 25–28.

Dundee, J. W. Current views on the clinical pharmacology of the barbiturates. *International Anesthesiology Clinics*, 1969, **7**, 3–29.

Dundee, J. W., McCleery, W. N. C., & McLoughlin, G. The hazard of thiopental anaesthesia in porphyria. *Anesthesia and Analgesia: Current Researches*, 1962, **41**, 567–574.

Dundee, J. W., & Wyant, G. M. *Intravenous anaesthesia.* Edinburgh, Scotland: Churchill Livingstone, 1974.

Einstein, S., & Garitano, W. Treating the drug abuser: Problems, factors, and alternatives. *International Journal of the Addictions*, 1972, **7**, 321–331.

Essig, C. F. Addiction to nonbarbiturate sedative and tranquilizing drugs. *Clinical Pharmacology and Therapeutics,* 1964, **5,** 334–343.

Essig, C. F., & Carter, W. W. Failure of diphenylhydantoin in preventing barbiturate withdrawal convulsions in dogs. *Neurology,* 1962, **12,** 481–484.

Essig, C. F., & Fraser, H. F. Failure of chlorpromazine to prevent barbiturate withdrawal convulsions. *Clinical Pharmacology and Therapeutics,* 1966, **7,** 466–469.

Evans, J. I., Lewis, S. A., Gibb, I. A. M., & Cheetham, M. Sleep and barbiturates: Some experiments and observations. *British Medical Journal,* 1968, **4,** 291–293.

Finkle, S. Ubiquitous reds: A local perspective on secobarbital abuse. *Clinical Toxicology,* 1971, **4,** 253–264.

Fischer, E., & Dilthey, A. Ueber C-Dialkylbarbitursäuern und über die Ureïde der Dialkylessigsäuren. *Justus Liebig's Annalen der Chemie,* 1904, **335,** 334–368.

Fischer, E., & von Mering, J. Ueber eine neue Classe von Schlafmitteln. *Die Therapie der Gegenwart,* 1903, **44,** 97–101.

Fitch, R. H. An experimental study of tolerance to barbiturates. *Journal of Pharmacology and Experimental Therapeutics,* 1930, **39,** 266–267.

Food and Drug Administration. Anticonvulsant linked with birth defect risk. *FDA Drug Bulletin,* July 1974.

Fraser, H. F., Shaver, M. R., Maxwell, E. S., Isbell, H., & Wikler, A. Fatal termination of barbiturate abstinence syndrome in man. *Journal of Pharmacology and Experimental Therapeutics,* 1952, **106,** 387.

Freeman, J. M. Neonatal seizures—diagnosis and management. *Journal of Pediatrics,* 1970, **77,** 701–708.

Garattini, S., Mussini, E., & Randall, L. O. (Eds.). *The benzodiazepines.* New York: Raven Press, 1973.

Gaspar, M. R., & Hare, R. R. Gangrene due to intra-arterial injection of drugs by drug addicts. *Surgery,* 1972, **72,** 573–577.

Geissler, W. Luminal, a new strongly acting hypnotic which may be given subcutaneously. *Munchener Medizinische Wochenschrift,* 1912, **59,** 922–924.

Gerhartz. Ueber einen Fall von Veronalvergiftung. *Berliner Klinische Wochenschrift,* 1903, **40,** 928.

Goldbaum, L. R., & Smith, P. K. The interaction of barbiturates with serum albumin and its possible relation to their disposition and pharmacological actions. *Journal of Pharmacology and Experimental Therapeutics,* 1954, **111,** 197–209.

Goldman, D. H., & Ulett, G. A. *Practical psychiatry for the internist.* St. Louis, Mo.: C. V. Mosby, 1968.

Grinker, R. R., & Spiegel, J. P. *War neuroses.* New York: Blakiston, McGraw-Hill, 1945.

Halleck, S. L. *The politics of therapy.* New York: Science House, 1971.

Hamburger, E. Barbiturate use in narcotic addicts. *Journal of the American Medical Association,* 1964, **189,** 366–368.

Hansch, C., & Clayton, J. Lipophilic character and biological activity of drugs. II: The parabolic case. *Journal of Pharmaceutical Sciences,* 1973, **62,** 1–21.

Hansten, P. D. *Drug interactions: Clinical significance of drug-drug interactions and drug effects on clinical laboratory results.* Philadelphia: Lea & Febiger, 1972.

Hauptmann, A. Luminal bei epilepsie. *Munchener Medizinische Wochenschrift,* 1912, **59,** 1907–1909.

Hinton, J. M. A comparison of the effects of six barbiturates and a placebo on insomnia and motility in psychiatric patients. *British Journal of Pharmacology,* 1963, **20,** 319–325.

Hirsch, R., & Imhof, J. E. A family therapy approach to the treatment of drug abuse and addiction. *Journal of Psychedelic Drugs,* 1975, **7**(2), 181–185.

Hofvendahl, A. Die bekämpfung der cocainvergiftung im tierversuch. *Biochemie Zeitschrift,* 1921, **117,** 55–66.

Hollister, L. Antianxiety drugs in clinical practice. In S. Garattini, E. Mussini, & L. O. Randall (Eds.), *The benzodiazepines.* New York: Raven Press, 1973.

Hollister, L. E., Bennett, J. L., Kimbell, I., Savage, C., & Overall, J. E. Diazepam in newly admitted schizophrenics. *Diseases of the Nervous System,* 1963, **24,** 746–750.

Hollister, L. E., Motzenbecker, F. P., & Degan, R. O. Withdrawal reactions from chlordiazepoxide ("librium"). *Psychopharmacologia,* 1961, **2,** 63–68.

Horsley, J. S. Narco-analysis. *Journal of Mental Science,* 1936, **82,** 416–422.

Howard, J., & Borges, P. Needle sharing in the Haight: Some social and psychological functions. *Journal of Psychedelic Drugs,* 1971, **4**(1), 71–80.

Ideström, C-M., & Cadenius, B. Chlordiazepoxide, dipiperon and amobarbital: Dose effect studies on human beings. *Psychopharmacologia,* 1963, **4,** 235–246.

Impens, E. The pharmacology of phenylethyl barbituric acid. *Deutsche Medizinische Wochenschrift,* **38,** 1912, 945–947. (Abstract: *Chemical Abstracts,* 1912, 2109.)

Isbell, H. Manifestations and treatment of addiction to narcotic drugs and barbiturates. *Medical Clinics of North America,* 1950, **34,** 425–438.

Jaffe, J. H. Drug addiction and drug abuse. In L. S. Goodman & A. Gilman (Eds.). *The pharmacological basis of therapeutics* (5th ed.), New York: Macmillan, 1975.

Jansson, B. Drug automatism as a cause of pseudo suicide. *Postgraduate Medicine,* 1961, **30**, A34-A40.

Judd, L. L., & Grant, I. Brain dysfunction in chronic sedative users. *Journal of Psychedelic Drugs,* 1975, **7**(2), 143–149.

Juliusberger, O. Dial-ciba, a new sedative and hypnotic. *Berliner Klinische Wochenschrift,* 1914, 643–645.

Juliusberger, O. Über Luminal, ein neues hypnoticum und sedativum. *Berliner Klinische Wochenschrift,* 1912, 940–942.

Jørgensen, J., & With, T. K. Acute porphyria. *Lancet,* 1947, **252**, 54–56.

Kales, A., Bixler, E. O., Tan, T-L., Scharf, M. B., & Kales, J. D. Chronic hypnotic drug use. Ineffectiveness, drug-withdrawal insomnia, and dependence. *Journal of the American Medical Association,* 1974, **227**, 513–517.

Kales, A., Jacobson, A., Kales, J. D., Marusak, C., & Hanley, J. Effects of drugs on sleep (noludar, doriden, nembutal, chloral hydrate, benadryl). *Psychophysiology,* 1968, **4**, 391–392.

Kales, A., Preston, T. A., Tan, T-L., & Allen, C. Hypnotics and altered sleep-dream patterns: I. All-night EEG studies of glutethimide, methyprylon, and pentobarbital. *Archives of General Psychiatry,* 1970, **23**, 211–218.

Kales, A., Preston, T., Tan, T-L., Scharf, M., & Kales, J. Effects of chronic hypnotic use. *Psychophysiology,* 1969, **6**, 259.

Kalinowsky, L. B. Convulsions in nonepileptic patients on withdrawal of barbiturates, alcohol and other drugs. *Archives of Neurology and Psychiatry,* 1942, **48**, 946–956.

Kaufman, A., Brickner, P. W., Varner, R., & Mashburn, W. Tranquilizer control. *Journal of the American Medical Association,* 1972, **221**, 1504–1506.

Klaesi, J. Über die therapeutische Anwendung, der "Dauernarkose" mittels Somnifens bei schizophrenen. *Zeitschrift für die Gesamte Neurologie und Psychiatrie,* 1922, **74**, 557–592.

Klein, D. F., & Davis, J. M. *Diagnosis and drug treatment of psychiatric disorders.* Baltimore: Williams & Wilkins, Co., 1969.

Kress. Veronalismus. *Therapeutische Monatshefte,* 1905, **19**, 467–471.

Laehr, H. Ein Fall von akuter Psychose nach chronischem Veronalgebrauch. *Allgemeine Zeitschrift für Psychiatrie,* 1912, **69**, 529–567.

Lasagna, L. A study of hypnotic drugs in patients with chronic diseases: Comparative efficacy of placebo; methyprylon (noludar); meprobamate (Miltown, Equanil); pentobarbital; phenobarbital; secobarbital. *Journal of Chronic Diseases*, 1956, **3**, 122–133.

Lennard, H. L., Epstein, L. J., Bernstein, A., & Ransom, D. C. *Mystification and drug misuse*. San Francisco: Jossey-Bass, 1971.

Lilienfeld, A. Veronal, ein neues Schlafmittel. *Berliner Klinische Wochenschrift*, 1903, **40**, 474–475.

Locket, S., & Angus, J. Poisoning by barbiturates: Success of conservative treatment. *Lancet*, 1952, **1**, 580.

Loewe, S. Clinical procedures with Luminal. *Deutch Medizinische Wochenschrift*, 1912, **38**, 947–948. (Abstract: *Chemical Abstracts*, 1912, 2110–2111.)

Long, R. H. Barbiturates, automatism and suicide. *Postgraduate Medicine*, 1960, **28**, A56–A72.

Loomis, T. A., & West, T. C. Comparative sedative effects of a barbiturate and some tranquilizer drugs on normal subjects. *Journal of Pharmacology and Experimental Therapeutics*, 1958, **122**, 525–531.

Luce, H., & Feigl, J. Über Luminalexantheme, zugleich ein Beitrag zur Behandlung der Chorea infantum. *Therapeutische Monatshefte*, 1918, **32**, 236–239.

Lundy, J. S. Intravenous anesthesia: Preliminary report of the use of two new thiobarbitures. *Proceedings of the Staff Meetings of the Mayo Clinic*, 1935, **10**, 536–543.

Lundy, J. S., & Osterberg, A. E. Review of the literature on the derivatives of barbituric acid. Chemistry; pharmacology; clinical use. *Proceedings of the Staff Meetings of the Mayo Clinic*, 1929, **4**, 386–416.

Marcus, J. B. Transcendental meditation: Consciousness expansion as an antidote to drug abuse. *Journal of Psychedelic Drugs*, 1975, **7**(2), 169–179.

Maurer, H. M., Wolff, J. A., Finster, G., Poppers, P. J., Pantuck, E., Kuntzman, R., & Conney, A. H. Reduction in concentration of total serum-bilirubin in offspring of women treated with phenobarbitone during pregnancy. *Lancet*, 1968, **2**, 122–124.

Menninger, W. C. Skin eruptions with phenobarbital (Luminal®). *Journal of the American Medical Association*, 1928, **9**, 14–18.

Meyer, H. J. Uber chronischen Schlafmittelmissbrauch und Phanodorm-psychosen. *Psychiatrisch-Neurologische Wochenschrift*, 1939, **41**, 275–281.

Meyer, R., & Rollet, M. Barbituric acid and barbiturates. In R. E. Kirk & D. F. Othmer (Eds.) *Encyclopedia of chemical technology*. Vol. 3 (2nd ed.). New York: John Wiley & Sons, 1964.

National Commission on Marijuana and Drug Abuse. *Drug use in America: Problem in perspective*. Report No. 2. Washington, D. C.: U.S. Government Printing Office, 1973.

Neuvonen, P. J., & Penttilä, O. Interaction between doxycycline and barbiturates. *British Medical Journal,* 1974, **1,** 535–536.

O'Neil v. State of New York, 323 N.Y.S. 2d 56, N.Y. Ct. of Claims, July 6, 1971.

Ormsby, H. B. Veronal dermatitis: Report of a case. *Cleveland Medical Journal,* 1908, **7,** 19–21.

Oswald, I., & Priest, R. G. Five weeks to escape the sleeping-pill habit. *British Medical Journal,* 1965, **2,** 1093–1095.

Palmer, H. D., & Braceland, F. J. Six years experience with narcosis therapy in psychiatry. *American Journal of Psychiatry,* 1937, **94,** 37–53.

Palmer, H. D., & Paine, A. L. Prolonged narcosis as therapy in the psychoses. *American Journal of Psychiatry,* 1932, **89,** 143–164.

Park, D. V. Biochemistry of the barbiturates. In H. Matthew (Ed.), *Acute Barbiturate Poisoning.* Amsterdam: Excerpta Medica, 1971.

Poole, A. K. Drug reactions from barbital (Veronal) and phenobarbital (Luminal). *Yale Journal of Biology and Medicine,* 1929, **1,** 345–351.

Reed, C. E., Driggs, M. F., & Foote, C. C. Acute barbiturate intoxication: A study of 300 cases based on a physiologic system of classification of the severity of the intoxication. *Annals of Internal Medicine,* 1952, **37,** 290–303.

Richards, R. A symptom of poisoning by hypnotics of the barbituric acid group. *British Medical Journal,* 1934, **1,** 331.

Rickels, K. Predictors of response to benzodiazepines in anxious outpatients. In S. Garattini, E. Mussini & L. O. Randall (Eds.), *The benzodiazepines.* New York: Raven Press, 1973.

Rising, M., & Stieglitz, J. The preparation of phenylethylbarbituric acid. *Journal of the American Chemical Society,* 1918, **40,** 723–730.

Seevers, M. H., & Tatum, A. L. Chronic experimental barbital poisoning. *Journal of Pharmacology and Experimental Therapeutics,* 1931, **42,** 217–231.

Senay, E. C., & Renault, P. F. Treatment methods for heroin addicts: A review. *Journal of Psychedelic Drugs,* 1971, **3,** 47–54.

Sexton, D. L., Pike, G. M., & Nielson, A. Exfoliative dermatitis and death due to phenobarbital. *Journal of the American Medical Association,* 1941, **116,** 700–701.

Shonle, H. A., Keltch, A. K., & Swanson, E. E. Dialkyl barbituric acids. *Journal of the American Chemical Society,* 1930, **52,** 2440–2451.

Shonle, H. A., & Moment, A. Some new hypnotics of the barbituric acid series. *Journal of the American Chemical Society,* 1923, **45,** 243–249.

Skinner, H. A. *The origins of medical terms.* New York: Hafner Publishing, 1970.

Smith, G. M., & Beecher, H. K. Amphetamine, secobarbital, and athletic performance: III.Quantitative effects on judgment. *Journal of the American Medical Association*, 1960, **172**, 1623–1629.

Smith, D. E., & Wesson, D. R. *Diagnosis and treatment of adverse reactions to sedative-hypnotics.* [DHEW Publication No. (ADM) 75–144.] Washington, D.C.: U.S. Government Printing Office, 1974.

Smith, D. E., & Wesson, D. R. Legitimate and illegitimate distribution of amphetamines and barbiturates. In D. E. Smith & D. R. Wesson. (Eds.), *Uppers and downers.* Englewood Cliffs, N.J.: Prentice-Hall, 1973.

Smith, D. E., & Wesson, D. R. A new method for treatment of barbiturate dependence. *Journal of the American Medical Association*, 1970, **213**, 294–295.

Smith, D. E., Wesson, D. R., & Lannon, R. New developments in barbiturate abuse. In *Drug abuse papers.* Berkeley: University of California, 1969.

Smith, D. E., Wesson, D. R., & Lerner, S. E. Treatment of the polydrug abuser in San Francisco with discussion of youth and polydrug abuse. Paper presented at the International Congress on Drug Abuse, Jerusalem, Israel, August 1974.

Stanton, E. M. Addiction and tolerance to barbiturates? The effects of daily administration and abrupt withdrawal of phenobarbital-sodium and pentobarbital-sodium in the albino rat. *Journal of Pharmacology and Experimental Therapeutics*, 1936, **57**, 245–252.

Subcommittee to Investigate Juvenile Delinquency. *Barbiturate Abuse—1971–1972.* Investigative and legislative hearings on barbiturate abuse, Committee on the Judiciary, U.S. Senate. Washington, D.C.: U.S. Government Printing Office, 1972.

Swanson, L. A., & Okada, T. Death after withdrawal of meprobamate. *Journal of the American Medical Association*, 1963, **184**, 780–781.

Swanson, E. E., Weaver, H. M., & Chen, K. K. Repeated administration of amytal. *American Journal of Mental Science*, 1937, **193**, 246–251.

Szasz, T. *Ceremonial chemistry.* Garden City, N.Y.: Anchor Press, 1974.

Tabern, D. L., & Volwiler, E. H. Sulfur-containing barbiturate hypnotics. *Journal of American Chemical Society*, 1935, **57**(2): 1961–1963.

Tatum, A. L. The present status of the barbiturate problem. *Physiological Reviews*, 1939, **19**, 472–502.

Tatum, A. L., Atkinson, A. J., & Collins, K. H. Acute cocain [sic] poisoning: Preliminary report of an experimental study. *Journal of the American Medical Association*, 1925, **84**, 1177.

Vallery-Radot, P., & Blamoutier, P. Accidents cutanéo-muqueux provoqués chez la même malade par le véronal et par un autre produit de la série barbiturique. *Société Médicale des Hopitaux de Paris Bulletin et Memoires*, 1925, **2**, 1382–1385.

Wain, H. *The story behind the work: Some interesting origins of medical terms.* Springfield, Ill.: Charles C Thomas, 1958.

Weinstein, E. A., & Malitz, S. Changes in symbolic expression with amytal sodium. *American Journal of Psychiatry*, 1954, **111**, 198–206.

Welton, D. G. Exfoliative dermatitis and hepatitis due to phenobarbital. *Journal of the American Medical Association*, 1950, **143**, 232–234.

Wesseling, H. Comparative study of the efficacy of diazepam, pentobarbital, and fentanyl-droperidol (Thalamonal®) against toxicity induced by local anesthetics in mice. In S. Garattini, E. Mussini & L. O. Randall (Eds.). *The benzodiazepines* New York: Raven Press, 1973.

Wesson, D. R., Gay, G. R., & Smith, D. E. Clinical-political issues of barbiturate use and abuse. *Contemporary Drug Problems*, 1972, 453–465.

Wesson, D. R., & Smith, D. E. A conceptual approach to detoxification. *Journal of Psychedelic Drugs*, 1974, **6**(2), 161–168.

Wikler, A. Diagnosis and treatment of drug dependence of the barbiturate type. *American Journal of Psychiatry*, 1955, **125**, 1–13.

Wikler, A. Diagnosis and treatment of drug dependence of the barbiturate type. *American Journal of Psychiatry*, 1968, **125**, 758–765.

Wikler, A., Fraser, H. F., Isbell, H., & Pescor, F. T. Electroencephalograms during cycles of addiction to barbiturates in man. *Electroencephalography and Clinical Neurophysiology*, 1955, **7**, 1–13.

Winstead, D. K., Anderson, A., Eilers, M. K., Blackwell, B., & Zaremba, A. L. Diazepam on demand: Drug-seeking behavior in psychiatric inpatients. *Archives of General Psychiatry*, 1974, **30**, 349–351.

Winter, C. A. The potentiating effect of antihistaminic drugs upon the sedative action of barbiturates. *Journal of Pharmacology and Experimental Therapeutics*, 1948, **94**, 7–11.

Wolpe, J. *The practice of behavior therapy.* New York: Pergamon Press, 1969.

Wulff, M. H. The barbiturate withdrawal syndrome: A clinical and electroencephalographic study. *Electroencephalography and Clinical Neurophysiology*, 1959, **14** (Suppl.).

Yaffe, S. J., Levy, G., Matsuzawa, T., & Baliah, T. Enhancement of glucuronide-conjugating capacity in a hyperbilirubinemic infant due to apparent enzyme induction by phenobarbital. *New England Journal of Medicine*, 1966, **275**, 1461–1466.

BIBLIOGRAPHY

Anderson, B. M., & Essex, H. E. Analysis of blood for certain barbiturates and the variability of their concentration in the blood. *Anesthesiology*, 1943, **4**, 113–125.

Armitage, G. H., & Sim, M. Barbiturate addiction and sensitivity. *British Journal of Medical Psychology*, 1960, **33**, 149.

Bain, J. A. Enzymatic aspects of barbiturate action. *Federation Proceedings*, 1952, **11**, 653–658.

Barraclough, B. M. Are there safer hypnotics than barbiturates? *Lancet*, 1974, **1**, 57.

Barsa, J. A., & Kline, N. S. Use of meprobamate in the treatment of psychotic patients. *American Journal of Psychiatry*, 1956, **112**, 1023.

Belleville, R. E., & Fraser, H. F. Tolerance to some effects of barbiturates. *Journal of Pharmacology and Experimental Therapeutics*, 1957, **120**, 469–474.

Brazier, M. A. *Brain mechanisms and consciousness*. Oxford, England: Blackwell, 1954.

Brodie, B. B. Physiological disposition and chemical fate of thiobarbiturates in the body. *Federation Proceedings*, 1952, **11**, 632–639.

Brodwall, E., & Stöa, K. F. A study of barbiturate clearance. *Acta Medica Scandinavica*, 1956, **154**, 139–144.

Brownstein, S. R., & Pacella, B. L. Convulsions following abrupt withdrawal of barbiturate: Clinical and electroencephalographic studies. *Psychiatric Quarterly*, 1943, **17**, 112–122.

Butler, T. C. Metabolic oxidation of phenobarbital to p-hydroxyphenobarbital. *Science*, 1954, **120**, 494.

Butler, T. C., Mahaffee, C., & Waddell, W. J. Phenobarbital: Studies of elimination, accumulation, tolerance, and dosage schedules. *Journal of Pharmacology and Experimental Therapeutics*, 1954, **111**, 425–435.

Chambers, C. D., & Moldestad, M. The evolution of concurrent opiate and sedative abuse in the United States. In J. C. Ball & C. D. Chambers (Eds.), *Epidemiology of opiate addiction in the United States*. Springfield, Ill.: Charles C. Thomas, 1970.

Clutton-Brock, J. Pain and the barbiturates. *Anaesthesia,* 1961, **16,** 80–88.

Cobb, S., & Miles, H. H. W. Symptoms due to withdrawal of barbiturates. *American Practitioner and Digest of Treatment,* 1951, **2,** 768–771.

Cochran, W. G., & Cox, G. M. *Experimental designs.* New York: John Wiley & Sons, 1950.

Cohen, S. The psychopharmacology of amphetamine and barbiturate dependence. In J. R. Wittenborn et al. (Eds.), *Drugs and youth.* Springfield, Ill.: Charles 'C. Thomas, 1970.

Conney, A. H. Pharmacological implications of microsomal enzyme induction. *Pharmacological Reviews,* 1967, **19,** 317, 366.

Crigler, J. F., & Gold, N. I. Sodium phenobarbital-induced decrease in serum bilirubin in an infant with congenital nonhemolytic jaundice and kernicterus. *Journal of Clinical Investigation,* 1966, **45,** 998–999.

Doran, W. J. Barbituric acid hypnotics. In F. F. Blick & H. Cox (Eds.), *Medicinal chemistry.* Vol. 4. New York: John Wiley & Sons, 1959.

Dox, A. W., & Hjort, A. M. The relative physiological properties of certain trialkyl and dialkyl barbituric acids. *Journal of Pharmacology and Experimental Therapeutics,* 1927, **31,** 455–472.

Dripps, R. D. Selective utilization of barbiturates as illustrated by a study of butabarbital (N.N.R.). *Journal of the American Medical Association,* 1949, **139,** 148–150.

Dunning, H. S. Convulsions following withdrawal of sedative medication. *New International Clinics,* 1940, **3,** 254–264.

Essig, C. F. Addiction to barbiturate and nonbarbiturate sedative drugs. In A. Wikler (Ed.), *The addictive states.* New York: Williams & Wilkins, 1968.

Essig, C. F. Clinical and experimental aspects of barbiturate withdrawal convulsions. *Epilepsia,* 1967, **8,** 21–30. (4th series.)

Essig, C. F. Withdrawal convulsions in dogs following chronic meprobamate intoxication. *Archives of Neurology and Psychiatry,* 1958, **80,** 414–417.

Ewing, J. A., & Bakewell, W. E. Diagnosis and management of depressant drug dependence. *American Journal of Psychiatry,* 1967, **123,** 909–917.

Ewing, J. A., & Haizlip, T. M. A controlled study of the habit forming propensities of meprobamate. *American Journal of Psychiatry,* 1958, **114,** 835.

Expert Committee on Addiction-Producing Drugs. *World Health Organization Technical Report Series,* No. 273, 1964.

Flynn, E. J., & Spector, S. Determination of barbiturate derivatives by radioimmunoassay. *Journal of Pharmacology and Experimental Therapeutics,* 1972, **181,** 547–554.

Fraser, H. F., Isbell, H., Eisenman, A. J., Wikler, A., & Pescor, F. T. Chronic barbiturate intoxication. *Archives of Internal Medicine*, 1954, **94**, 34–41.

Fraser, H. F., Shaver, M. R., Maxwell, E. S., & Isbell, H. Death due to withdrawal of barbiturates. *Annals of Internal Medicine*, 1953, **38**, 1319–1325.

Fraser, H. F., Wikler, A., Essig, C. F., & Isbell, H. Degree of physical dependence induced by secobarbital or pentobarbital. *Journal of the American Medical Association*, 1958, **166**, 126–129.

Freedman, A. M., & Kaplan, H. I. (Eds.). *Comprehensive textbook of psychiatry.* Baltimore: Williams & Wilkins, 1967.

Gardner, A. J. Withdrawal fits in barbiturate addicts. *Lancet*, 1967, **2**, 337–338.

Goldstein, A. A pharmacology teaching exercise with barbiturates. *Journal of Medical Education*, 1953, **28**, 48–50.

Goodman, L. S., & Gillman, A. (Eds.). *The pharmacological basis of therapeutics.* (5th ed.) New York: Macmillan, 1975.

Gruber, C. M., Ellis, F. W., & Freedman, G. A toxicological and pharmacological investigation of sodium sec-butyl ethyl barbituric acid (butisol sodium). *Journal of Pharmacology and Experimental Therapeutics*, 1944, **81**, 254–268.

Hadden, J., Johnson, K., Smith, S., Price, L., & Giardina, E. Acute barbiturate intoxication: Concepts of management. *Journal of the American Medical Association*, 1969, **209**, 893–900.

Hartmann, E. L. *The functions of sleep.* New Haven, Conn.: Yale University Press, 1973.

Heldt, T. J. Therapeutic use of prolonged sodium amytal narcosis. *American Journal of Psychiatry*, 1947, **104**, 27–35.

Hewitt, R. T. A psychosis with barbiturate withdrawal. *Journal of Nervous and Mental Disease*, 1950, **112**, 526–530.

Hill, H. E., & Belleville, R. E. Effects of chronic barbiturate intoxication on motivation and muscular coordination. *Archives of Neurology and Psychiatry*, 1953, **70**, 180–188.

Hunter, R. A., & Greenberg, H. P. Barbiturate addiction simulating spontaneous hyperinsulinism. *Lancet*, 1954, **2**, 58–62.

Hunter, R. A., Merivale, W. H. H., & Smith, A. J. Disturbances of carbohydrate metabolism caused by barbiturates and alcohol. *Lancet*, 1955, **2**, 1353–1355.

Hussey, H. H. Drug automatism: A myth. *Journal of the American Medical Association*, 1974, **230**, 265.

Irey, N. S., & Froede, R. C. Evaluation of deaths from drug overdose:
• A clinicopathologic study. *American Journal of Clinical Pathology*, 1974, **61**, 778–784.

Isbell, H. Abuse of barbiturates. *Journal of the American Medical Association,* 1956, **162,** 660–661.

Isbell, H. Addiction to barbiturates and the barbiturate abstinence syndrome. *Annals of Internal Medicine,* 1950, **33,** 108–121.

Isbell, H., Altschul, S., Kornetsky, C. H., Eisenman, A. J., Flanary, H. G., & Fraser, H. F. Chronic barbiturate intoxication: An experimental study. *Archives of Neurology and Psychiatry,* 1950, **64,** 1–28.

Isbell, H., & Fraser, H. F. Addiction to analgesics and barbiturates. *Pharmacological Reviews,* 1950, **2,** 355–397.

Isbell, H., & White, W. M. Clinical characteristics of addictions. *American Journal of Medicine,* 1953, **14,** 558–565.

James, I. P. Drug-withdrawal psychoses. *American Journal of Psychiatry,* 1963, **119,** 880–881.

Jansson, B. A catamnestic study of 476 attempted suicides. *Acta Psychiatry Scand,* 1962, **38,** 183–198.

Kales, A. (Ed.). *Sleep. Physiology & Pathology: A Symposium.* Philadelphia: J. B. Lippincott, 1969.

Knoefel, P. K., Herwick, R. P., & Loevenhart, A. S. The prevention of acute intoxication from certain local anesthetics. *Journal of Pharmacology and Experimental Therapeutics,* 1928, **33,** 265.

Kolb, L. Drug addiction: A study of some medical cases. *Archives of Neurology and Psychiatry,* 1928, **20,** 171–183.

Kornetsky, C. H. Psychological effects of chronic barbiturate intoxication. *Archives of Neurology and Psychiatry,* 1951, **65,** 557–567.

Kubie, L. S., & Margolin, S. The therapeutic role of drugs in the process of repression, dissociation and synthesis. *Psychosomatic Medicine,* 1945, **7,** 147–151.

Langrod, J. *Multiple drug use among heroin users.* New York: Bureau of Applied Social Research, Columbia University, 1969.

Lasagna, L. A comparison of hypnotic agents. *Journal of Pharmacology and Experimental Therapeutics,* 1954, **111,** 9–20.

Lemere, F. Drug habitation. *Journal of the American Medical Association,* 1956, **160,** 1431.

Lipton, E. L. The amytal interview: A review. *American Practitioner and Digest of Treatment,* 1950, **1,** 148–163.

Loomis, T. A., & West, T. C. The influence of alcohol on automobile driving ability: An experimental study for the evaluation of certain medicolegal aspects. *Quarterly Journal of Studies on Alcohol,* 1958, **19,** 30–46.

Lous, P. Plasma levels and urinary excretion of three barbituric acids after oral administration to man. *Acta Pharmacologica et Toxicologica,* 1954, **10,** 147–165.

Malamud, W. *American psychiatry 1844–1944.* New York: Columbia University Press, 1944.

Manning, D. E., Stout, A. G., & Zemp, J. W. Effects of maternal pheno-barbital administration on some aspects of neonatal brain development. *Federation Proceedings*, 1971, **30**, 495.

Maynert, E. W. The distribution and fate of dialkylbarbiturates. *Federation Proceedings*, 1952, **11**, 625–631.

Maynert, E. W., & Van Dyke, H. B. The metabolism of barbiturates. *Pharmacological Reviews*, 1949, **1**, 217–242.

McGeachy, T. E., & Bloomer, W. E. The phenobarbital sensitivity syndrome. *American Journal of Medicine*, 1953, **14**, 600–604.

McKenzie, R. E., & Elliott, L. L. Effects of secobarbital and d-amphetamine on performance during a simulated air mission. *Aerospace Medicine*, 1965, **36**, 774–779.

Myers, F. H., Jawetz, E., and Goldfien, A. (Eds.). *Review of medical pharmacology.* Los Altos, Calif.: Lange, 1968.

Mitcheson, M., Davidson, J., Hawks, D., Hitchins, L., & Malone, S. Sedative abuse by heroin addicts. *Lancet*, 1970, 1(7647), 606–607.

Mulé, S. J. Detection and identification of drugs of dependence. In S. J. Mulé & H. Brill (Eds.). *Clinical and biological aspects of drug dependence.* Cleveland, Ohio: CRC Press, 1972.

Mulé, S. J., Bastos, M. L., Jukofsky, D., & Saffer, E. Routine identification of drugs of abuse in human urine: II. Development and application of the XAD-2 resin column method. *Journal of Chromatography*, 1971, **63**, 289–301.

Mohr, R. C., & Mead, B. T. Meprobamate addiction. *New England Journal of Medicine*, 1958, **259**, 865–868.

National Clearinghouse for Drug Abuse Information and Donald R. Wesson Associates. *Amphetamine.* National Clearinghouse for Drug Abuse Information Report Series, No. 28. [DHEW Publication No. (ADM) 74–52] Rockville, Maryland, 1974.

Nyswander, M. *The drug addict as a patient.* New York: Grune & Stratton, 1956.

O'Donnell, J. A. The natural history of drug abuse. *Medical Arts and Sciences*, 1971, **25**, 3–14.

Osgood, C. W. Convulsive seizures following barbiturate withdrawal. *Journal of the American Medical Association*, 1947, **133**, 104–105.

Page, I. H., & Coryllos, P. Isoamyl ethyl barbituric acid (amytal) its use as an intravenous anesthetic. *Journal of Pharmacology and Experimental Therapeutics*, 1926, **27**, 189–200.

Parker, K. D., Elliott, H. W., Wright, J. A., Nomof, N., & Hine, C. H. Blood and urine concentrations of subjects receiving barbiturates, meprobamate, glutethimide, or diphenylhydantoin. *Clinical Toxicology*, 1970, **3**, 131–145.

Parsons, T. W. Clinical comparison of barbiturates as hypnotics. *British Medical Journal*, 1963, **4**, 1035–1037.

Pohlish, K., & Panse, F. *Schlafmittelsmissbrauch.* Leipzig: Georg Thieme, 1934.

Polakow, R. L., & Doctor, R. M. Treatment of marijuana and barbiturate dependency by contingency contracting. *Journal of Behavior Therapy and Experimental Psychiatry,* 1973, **4,** 375–377.

Raventós, J. The distribution in the body and metabolic fate of barbiturates. *Journal of Pharmacy and Pharmacology,* 1954, **6,** 217–235.

Ray, O. S. *Drugs, society, and human behavior.* St. Louis, Mo.: C. V. Mosby, 1972.

Reichard, J. D. Addiction: Some theoretical considerations as to its nature, cause, prevention and treatment. *American Journal of Psychiatry,* 1947, **103,** 721–730.

Reitan, R. M. The comparative effects of placebo, ultran, and meprobamate on psychologic test performances. *Antibiotic Medicine and Clinical Therapy,* 1957, **4,** 158–165.

Remmer, H. Tolerance to barbiturates by increased breakdown. In H. Steinberg (Ed.). *Scientific basis of drug dependence.* New York: Grune & Stratton, 1969.

Resnick, R. B., Kestenbaum, R., Gaztanaga, P., Volavka, J., & Freedman, A. M. Experimental techniques for rapid withdrawal from methadone maintenance: Results of pilot trials. Paper presented at the First National Drug Abuse Conference, Chicago, March 1974.

Richards, R. K., & Taylor, J. D. Some factors influencing distribution, metabolism and action of barbiturates: A review. *Anesthesiology,* 1956, **17,** 414–458.

Rutherdale, J. A., Medline, A., Sinclair, J. C., Buchner, B., & Olin, J. S. Hepatitis in drug users. *American Journal of Gastroenterology,* 1972, **58,** 275–287.

Sands, L. J. Barbital (veronal) intoxication. *Journal of the American Medical Association,* 1923, **81,** 1519–1521.

Schubert, H. Zur Frage des Schlafmittelmissbrauches. *Die Medizinische Welt,* 1937, **2,** 47–50.

Seevers, M. H. Abuse of barbiturates and amphetamines. *Postgraduate Medicine,* 1965, **37,** 45–51.

Shagass, C., Azima, H., & Sangowicz, J. Effect of meprobamate in sustained high dosage on the electroencephalogram and sedation threshold. *Electroencephalography and Clinical Neurophysiology,* 1959, **11,** 275–283.

Smith, D. E., & Wesson, D. R. Phenobarbital technique for treatment of barbiturate dependence. *Archives of General Psychiatry,* 1971, **24,** 56–60.

Smith, D. E., Wesson, D. R., & Lannon, R. A. New developments in barbiturate abuse. *Clinical Toxicology*, 1970, **3**, 57–65.

Stenchever, M. A., & Jarvis, J. A. Effect of barbiturates on the chromosomes of human cells in vitro—a negative report. *Journal of Reproductive Medicine*, 1970, **5**, 69–71.

Tatum, A. L., & Seevers, M. H. Theories of drug addiction. *Physiological Reviews*, 1931, **11**, 107–121.

Toman, J. E. P., & Christensen, E. K. Ethchlorvynol (placidyl) compared with secobarbital and pentobarbital for EEG sedation. *Federation Proceedings*, 1956, **15**, 492.

Tyson, R. M., Shrader, E. A., & Perlman, H. H. Drugs transmitted through breast milk: II. Barbiturates. *Journal of Pediatrics*, 1938, **13**, 86–90.

Wagner, C. P. Pharmacologic action of barbiturates: Their use in neuropsychiatric conditions. *Journal of the American Medical Association*, 1933, **101**, 1787–1791.

Waters, D. J. Intra-arterial thiopentone: A physico-chemical phenomenon. *Anaesthesia*, 1966, **21**, 346–356.

Willcox, W. H. Discussion on the use and abuse of hypnotics. *British Medical Journal*, 1913, **2**, 661–665.

Wesson, D. R., Gay, G. R., & Smith, D. E. Treatment techniques for narcotic withdrawal with special reference to mixed narcotic-sedative addictions. *Journal of Psychedelic Drugs*, 1971, 4(2), 118–122.

Work, P. Barbital (Veronal) addiction. *Archives of Neurology and Psychiatry*, 1928, **19**, 324–328.

Wright, J. T. The value of barbiturate estimations in the diagnosis and treatment of barbiturate intoxication. *Quarterly Journal of Medicine*, 1955, **24**, 95–108.

Ziskind, E., & Ziskind, E. S. Phenobarbital contraindicated in parkinsonism. *Journal of the American Medical Association*, 1937, **109**, 20–23.

INDEX

Alcohol: barbiturates and, 24, 34-35, 64, 74, 75; and disinhibition, 30*t*, 68-69; intoxication from, compared with barbiturate intoxication, 27; parameters of dependence and toleration for, 34*t*; secobarbital and, 58; sedative-hypnotics and, 101-102; withdrawal, use of diallylbarbituric acid for, 16

Allergy: to adulterants in intravenous barbiturates, 79; to barbiturates, 32

Amitriptyline, 70; and barbiturate withdrawal, 68

Amobarbital sodium: abuse, 54*f*; blood concentrations related to behavioral changes and, 29*t*; and coumarin anticoagulants, 37; in diagnosis of organic brain damage, 48; disinhibition euphoria produced by, 30*t*; federal controls on, 111-112; in narcotherapy, 47, 93; neuropsychiatric tests of subjective effects of, 27-28; phenobarbital withdrawal equivalent for, 99*t*; and secobarbital, *see* Secobarbital and amobarbital; synthesis of, 16

Amphetamine users: and barbiturates, 75-76; and motor performance studies, 27

Amytol. *See* Amobarbital sodium

Antibiotics, phenobarbital and, 37-38

Anticoagulants, interaction with barbiturates, 37

Antihistamines, barbiturates and, 38

Antipsychotics, causing coma and convulsions from overdose, 82*t*

Anxiety reduction, barbiturates and, 42-43

Aquachloral Supprettes. *See* Chloral hydrate

Arterial blood gases, determination of respiratory insufficiency and, 86, 87

Arteries, complications of barbiturate injection into, 76-79

Barbital: abuse, 52; binding to serum albumin, 24; and cocaine toxicity, 49-50; dermatitis, 32; sensitivity reactions to, 32; synthesis of, 15; withdrawal, 93-94

Barbiturate abuse: and aftercare, 104-107; attitudes of medical profession toward, 107; and availability of barbiturates, 107-108, 109*f*, 112; complications of, 73-90; decline in 53, 54*t*; distinguished from misuse, 54-57; extent of, 13-14; historical background, 52-53; nonmedical aspects of, 104-116; prevalence of, 53, 54*t*; social cost of, 112-114; solutions for, 115-116

Barbiturate intoxication: behavioral changes related to blood concentrations of barbiturates in, 28, 29*t*, 30; chronic, 33; episodic, 73-75; subjective effects of, 27-28, 29*t*, 30*t*; and user's expectations, 28

Barbiturate misuse: distinguished from abuse, 54-57; medical, 57-61; nonmedical, 61-66

Barbiturate overdose: and intravenous use, 75; and mixed drug overdose, 89; Reed system for estimating degree of, 87, 88*t*; and tissue necrosis, 89-90

Barbiturate toxicity: EEG and, 31*f*, 32; impaired functioning and, 26-27

Barbiturate use: assessment of motivation for, 66-72; episodic, sources of supply for, 74-75

Barbiturate withdrawal: detoxification procedures for, 95-99; signs and symptoms in infants and adults of, 100*t*; syndrome, 93-95; treatment strategies for, 95

Barbiturates: alcohol and, 24, 34-35, 64, 74, 75; amphetamines and, 75-76; antibiotics and, 37-38; as antidote to effects of other drugs, 49-50, 64-65; and antihistamines, 38; and anxiety reduction, 42-43; arterial injection of, 76-79; benefits of, 13; benzodiazepines as replacement for, 16, 114-115; binding to serum albumin, 24; CNS-active, 19*f*, 20; chronic use of, 33-36; classification of, 20-21, 22*t*-23*t*; convulsive properties of, 20; detection in biological fluids, 25-26; development of, 15-16; difference between nonmedical use and misuse of, 62; in differential diagnosis of schizophrenia and stuporous depressive states, 47-48; and diphenylhydantoin, 37, 98; disadvantages and advantages of, 114-115; dosage differential between mild toxicity and disinhibition, 97; Drug Enforcement Administration ruling on, 51; duration of effects of, 25; early uses for, 15-16; effects on central nervous system, 21, 24-32; as enzyme inducers, *see* Liver; in epilepsy treatment, 48, 50; forgetting taking of, *see* Drug automatism;